Sciatica and Chronic Pain

Robert W. Baloh

Sciatica and Chronic Pain

Past, Present and Future

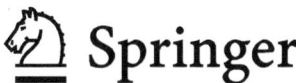 Springer

Robert W. Baloh, MD
Department of Neurology
University of California, Los Angeles
Los Angeles, CA, USA

ISBN 978-3-030-06741-0   ISBN 978-3-319-93904-9   (eBook)
https://doi.org/10.1007/978-3-319-93904-9

This Springer imprint is published by Springer Nature, under the registered company Springer Nature Switzerland AG
The registered company address is: Gewerbestrasse 11, 6330 Cham, Switzerland

Foreword

In *Sciatica and Chronic Pain: Past, Present and Future*, Professor Baloh addresses a common, universal problem directly related to man's upright posture. As such, it has afflicted man since prehistoric times. Our understanding of sciatica and pain has evolved over time. Modern imaging has contributed greatly to our appreciation of the relationships of nerve roots contributing to the sciatic nerve and the importance of adjacent structures of bone, cartilage, and disc. Our understanding of the phenomenon of pain and its physiology and chemistry is perhaps less complete. Management of patients with sciatica and chronic pain still poses a major challenge. Surprisingly, few have attempted to address this important problem.

Our perception of pain and response to pain is very individual and differs widely among people. *Sciatica and Chronic Pain: Past, Present and Future* delves into different aspects of pain from neural networks, neural transmitters, and genetic viewpoints and provides us with a glimpse of how various factors may interact to make us perceive pain. This book also provides a concise yet complete guide to the management of patients with sciatica. It explores the multifaceted approach to management of chronic pain from many viewpoints, including of course the pharmacological and surgical, as well as less orthodox approaches to pain. As such, it should be of interest to a wide audience, including students, physicians, as well as patients.

The historical perspectives are not only of interest but allow us to infer that our understanding of pain mechanisms will expand with current and future research, no doubt leading to even better methods of pain management.

Ulrich Batzdorf, MD
Professor of Neurosurgery
David Geffen School of Medicine at UCLA
Ronald Regan Medical Center
Los Angeles, CA, USA

Preface

I noticed a burning pain in my right buttock one Sunday morning. Since I frequently injured myself during my weekly tennis match on Saturday, at first I was not concerned. I tore my rotator cuff in the past and after surgical repair I could only play once a week without reinjuring the shoulder. But the pain gradually got worse and I noticed occasional sharp pains shooting into the outside of my right leg. I thought the pain might be coming from my hip possibly arthritis of the hip since my father had severe arthritis of the hip as he got older and I am a big believer in genetics. But when I saw the orthopedic surgeon who repaired my rotator cuff tear, he could not find anything wrong with my hip. We agreed that the pain was probably sciatica due to arthritis in my back and that I should lay off tennis and take ibuprofen as needed for the pain.

At least 5% of the general population suffers from sciatica and about 10% have some type of chronic neuropathic pain. Sciatica is the most common cause of chronic neuropathic pain, yet there is no consensus on how to manage this common painful disorder. Treatments developed thousands of years ago are still in common use. I am a professor of neurology at the University of California in Los Angeles and I have been teaching general neurology to medical students and neurology residents for more than four decades. I have treated many cases of sciatica over the years and I am well aware of the controversies regarding best treatments. In this book, I address the following questions from the point of view of a clinical neurologist, a teacher of neurology, and a person who has experienced sciatica.

- How is pain detected and perceived?
- What is sciatica and what are the causes?
- What are the treatment options for new onset sciatica?
- Why does the pain persist in many cases?
- What are the treatment options for chronic pain?
- And what new treatments are on the horizon?

The goal of the book is to provide a concise overview of sciatica and chronic pain. I have a longstanding interest in the history of medicine and I use historical context to set the stage for understanding new concepts. As in all areas of neuroscience and medicine, there is a "jargon" that goes with the field. I have attempted to minimize the impact of the jargon on understanding new concepts by defining terms as they are introduced. Charts, figures, and tables help clarify new concepts. Finally, three patients with sciatica and chronic pain are followed serially throughout the book to illustrate important concepts discussed in the text.

Robert W. Baloh, MD
Distinguished Professor of Neurology
David Geffin School of Medicine at UCLA
Ronald Regan Medical Center
Los Angeles, CA, USA

Acknowledgments

I thank my neurology colleagues Melissa Spencer and Leif Havton for reviewing early drafts of the book and providing helpful comments. I want to particularly thank Rick Batzdorf for his helpful suggestions and for writing the Foreword to the book. I thank Julie (Juhyun) Kim for drawing several of the figures and her patience in getting them just right. Julie is a nurse practitioner at Mount Sinai Hospital in New York and a talented young medical illustrator. My wife, Grace, provided helpful suggestions and constant support. Finally, I want to thank Michael Griffin and Richard Lansing at Springer for helping me get the book together.

Contents

Chapter 1
Introduction

Pain is unlike any other body sensation. Imagine having pain 24 h a day so that you never sleep soundly or do anything without being aware of pain. You take pain medication but the medication upsets your stomach and makes you feel "spacey," and yet the pain is still there. Or what if you had one of the rare genetic disorders where pain sensation does not develop such that you would not feel pain and would be in great danger of injuring yourself. Boiling an egg for breakfast could result in a third degree burn. Or you could fall asleep with your leg hanging over the side of a recliner, block the circulation to your leg, and without the normal warning pain, you could lose the leg.

Overview of Pain

Stated simply, pain is the body's defense system against noxious stimuli. Nerve endings in the skin and other organs sense the harmful stimuli and send signals (nerve impulses) to the spinal cord and brain for appropriate evasive actions, like pulling your hand away from a hot stove. But pain is much more than that: it activates primitive areas of the brain such as the limbic system that controls emotions such as fear, anger, and rage. On top of that, the meaning of pain depends greatly on your prior experience. A kind of "priming of the pump" occurs: if you have experienced severe pain in the past you can be incapacitated with just the anticipation of pain. And I think we can all agree that it is hard to have a good outlook on life when you live with constant pain.

How we perceive pain depends on many factors including genetic, environmental, cultural, and social. Although gene mutations that cause complete loss of pain sensation are rare, minor genetic variants in proteins involved in the development and function of pain pathways influence the differences in sensitivity to pain from individual to individual. Of course, the environment in which the pain occurs is also very important. Pain associated with a sudden injury such as a bone fracture or

© Springer International Publishing AG, part of Springer Nature 2019
R. W. Baloh, *Sciatica and Chronic Pain*,
https://doi.org/10.1007/978-3-319-93904-9_1

ligament tear is expected and tends to be better tolerated than the insidious onset of pain associated with an occult infection or tumor. Even though it is more intense, the sudden brief stabbing pain associated with sciatica is much better tolerated than the continuous deep aching, burning pain that often accompanies it.

Pain has different meanings in different cultures and in different social circumstances. In some cultures pain is synonymous with suffering whereas in others pain is considered a path to redemption. Whether one considers pain as punishment or a minor nuisance in the path to some greater good undoubtedly influences the perception of pain. For example, the pain experienced by a religious zealot who repeatedly flails himself with a whip for perceived sins against God is different than the pain experienced by a man receiving 50 lashes for stealing a loaf of bread to feed his family. Although excruciating, the pain of childbirth is cherished in some cultures where it is considered necessary for a successful delivery of a healthy child. In his book "Pain: a Cultural History", Spanish historian Javier Moscoso (2012), tells the story of a woman burned at the stake because she asked for pain relief during the birth of her child.

We feel our own pain but we also can "feel" the pain of others. The anterior cingulate cortex, an area of the cerebral cortex that is critical for processing pain signals, is activated when you look at photographs of another person experiencing pain. Furthermore, the amount of activity in the anterior cingulate cortex strongly correlates with one's perception of the severity of the other person's pain. Empathy for pain in others is not exclusive to humans or even primates as pain perception in mice is affected by observing pain in their cage mates.

Neuropathic Pain and Sciatica

Neuropathic pain is by far the worst kind of pain. Just about everyone has experienced the excruciating pain caused by damage to the nerve at the base of a tooth. Imagine undergoing a root canal without an anesthetic. A ruptured disc with sciatic nerve compression can make a stoic grown man scream out and cry like a baby. Post herpetic pain that occurs after herpes zoster infection of a nerve (shingles) can turn a contented senior into a depressed recluse. Although pain associated with diabetic neuropathy is less intense than most other nerve pain the constant unrelenting burning sensation can be unbearable.

Neuropathic pain results from damage to nerves. When acute, neuropathic pain serves as a warning signal that something is wrong so that you avoid activities that aggravate the pain and allow the nerve to heal. When chronic, neuropathic pain often serves no useful purpose and can become a disease in itself. The dividing line between acute and chronic pain, is arbitrarily set at 3 months. As a rule, acute neuropathic pain is associated with swelling, tenderness and muscle spasm at the site of the nerve injury due to inflammation. By contrast, chronic neuropathic pain is associated with overall increased sensitivity to pain due to reactive changes in nerve pain pathways.

Sciatica is the most common variety of neuropathic pain with a lifetime prevalence of at least 5%. It is not a disease, although for centuries medical practitioners have considered it as such. It's simply a pain in the leg usually starting in the back and radiating into the buttock and down the leg into the foot, following the sensory distribution of the sciatic nerve, the largest nerve in the body. It has many causes and can have many different characteristics from a constant dull ache to a lancinating shock-like sensation. It can come on suddenly after straining or lifting or it can develop gradually without any apparent trigger. As we will see later the triggers and the speed of onset are important in determining the cause.

Although people with sciatica often have associated back pain as a rule management of people with back pain alone is different from management of people with back pain and sciatica. Nearly everyone has experienced back pain at some time in life and back pain is chronic in up to 30% of the population. Most back pain is musculoskeletal in origin so managements focus on improving musculoskeletal function such as with heat, massage and stretching, whereas, sciatica is due to nerve damage so treatments focus on relieving or decreasing the effects of the nerve damage when possible. Some treatments used for back pain can actually aggravate sciatica. For example, certain types of physical therapy and chiropractic manipulations can increase nerve damage and worsen the pain. The most effective way to treat sciatica is to identify and treat the underlying cause. However, early on when the diagnosis is unclear, symptomatic treatment can provide pain relief until a diagnosis is clear or until the body heals itself.

Content of the Book

This book is divided into four parts: Chap. 2 provides an overview of how pain is detected and perceived; Chaps. 3 and 4 address the causes and management of new onset sciatica; Chaps. 5 and 6 cover imaging the back and the use of injections and surgery for treating sciatica; and Chaps. 7, 8, and 9 focus on chronic neuropathic pain addressing why the pain becomes chronic, current treatments and promising future treatments. There is a brief summary chapter at the end. Before addressing the causes and treatments for sciatica it is important to have a basic understanding of pain mechanisms. Chapter 2 uses historical perspective to provide a framework for understanding how pain is detected in the peripheral nervous system and how it is perceived in the brain. Chapters 3 and 4 summarize the logic for identifying the cause and appropriate management of new onset sciatica. Since the majority of people with new onset sciatica get better within 6 weeks regardless of the cause there is a general consensus that initial management should be conservative. A key component to the management strategy is to identify "red flags" that require immediate referral to a specialist and imaging of the back. By carefully watching for red flags listed in Table 3.1 one can decide on the best course of management. If sciatica worsens or does not improve within 6 weeks imaging of the back is recommended. Chapter 5 describes the methods for imaging the back, likely findings and pitfalls in interpreting the imaging results. When sciatica persists beyond 6 weeks it becomes critical to make a correct diagnosis and plan specific treatments outlined in Chap. 6. Anesthetic and steroid injections and surgical options are discussed in detail and the pros and cons for each procedure are presented for each disorder. Table 6.1 outlines the key information that patients need to know when contemplating back surgery for a herniated disc.

Sciatica becomes chronic in about a third of people who have new onset sciatica. Although the reasons why pain persists are not always clear, numerous well documented risk factors for developing chronic pain are discussed in Chap. 7. Repeat surgeries and regular use of pain medications play a surprising role in developing chronic sciatica. As a rule treatments of chronic pain outlined in Chap. 8 are completely different from treatments of acute sciatica. Treatments for chronic pain focus on stabilizing damaged nerves and decreasing central sensitization to pain. Although current medications can be effective, bothersome side effects are common since the medications have multiple actions in addition to pain control. Promising future treatments described in Chap. 9 target pain specific proteins and promise to be more effective with less overall side effects.

Suggested Additional Reading

Cervero F. Understanding pain. Cambridge, MA: The MIT Press; 2012.
Moscoso J. Pain: a cultural history. London: Palgrave Macmillan; 2012.

Chapter 2
Nerves and the Detection and Perception of Pain

Consider the problems facing very early investigators who were trying to understand how nerves were related to pain. On gross examination, nerves, tendons and ligaments all looked alike and the brain was a fragile gelatinous blob that easily fell apart. Initial theories on nerves and pain focused on supernatural forces such as animal spirits and souls. The famous Greek philosopher, Plato, recognized two different souls, the mortal soul responsible for pain, pleasure and lust, located in the liver and heart and the immortal soul responsible for rational behavior, located in the brain. Plato felt that pain acted exclusively on the mortal soul but it could alter the ability of the immortal soul to act rationally. Unlike Plato, his pupil Aristotle localized the immortal soul to the heart and believed that pain and pleasure resulted from ripples in the blood vessels of the heart.

Early Ideas on How Pain Was Detected

Rene Descartes, the seventeenth century French mathematician and philosopher provided the first detailed theory on pain transmission and nerves. Descartes expanded on the model of the famous Roman physician, Galen who considered nerves to be hollow tubes that carried mysterious "animal spirits" from the ventricles of the brain to activate muscles. To Descartes animal spirits were a "very fine air or wind" that inflated the ventricles like the sails of a ship are inflated by the wind. For reflex behavior such as withdrawal from a painful stimulus, he postulated that thin filaments within each nerve tube controlled tiny valves in the ventricles of the brain that in turn controlled the flow of animal spirits into the nerves (Fig. 2.1). Painful pressure or heat against the skin would move the filaments (like pulling on a rope to ring a bell), open the valves and release animal spirits from the ventricles into the nerve causing a reflex muscle contraction. The bulging of a muscle represented the influx of animal spirits.

© Springer International Publishing AG, part of Springer Nature 2019
R. W. Baloh, *Sciatica and Chronic Pain*,
https://doi.org/10.1007/978-3-319-93904-9_2

Fig. 2.1 Descartes illustrates reflex withdraw from a painful stimulus in his book, De Homine, published in 1662. Heat from the fire activates tiny filaments in the hollow nerve, opening pores in the ventricle (F), releasing animal spirits to inflate the muscles of the leg and withdrawal the foot from the fire

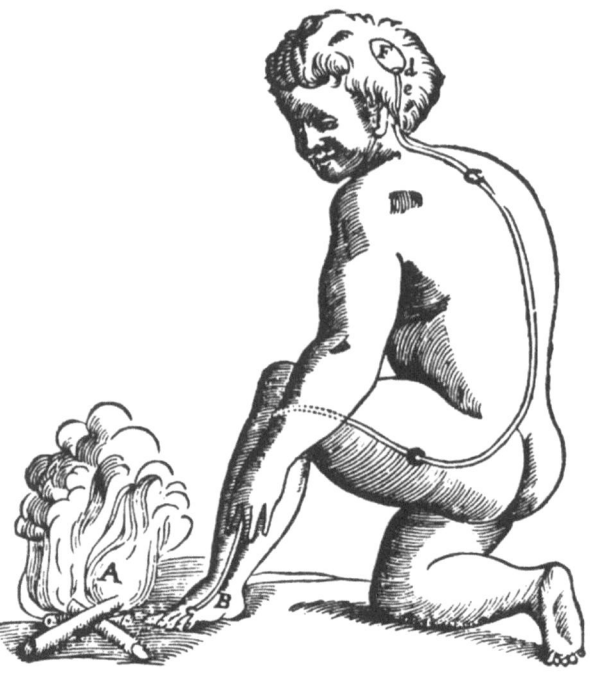

In Descartes' model, animal spirits were pumped into the ventricles of the brain by the heart and the ventricles pumped them back down the hollow nerves to inflate the muscles. Descartes was a philosopher not an anatomist. At the time Descartes published his famous book "Principes de la Philosophie" (Principles of Philosophy) in 1644 a young physician in Oxford England, Thomas Willis, was busily dissecting hundreds of animals and humans including many of his own patients who had died from brain diseases. When he looked at nerves under a magnifying glass he noted that they were solid cords not hollow tubes so he felt that they must contain very tiny pores for the animal spirits to move through. To Willis animal spirits represented a fundamental force derived from the soul that moved within nerves. He developed methods to remove and preserve the brain from the skull so that he could study it in detail. When he injected dye into the arteries supplying the brain he saw a rich network of arteries particularly at the base but none of the dye entered the ventricles as proposed by Descartes. Willis speculated that the brain itself not the ventricles must be the center for reflex and cognitive processes. Animal spirits arriving at the brain in sensory nerves were either reflected back down to the motor nerves of muscles to account for reflex behavior such as withdrawal of the hand from a painful stimulus or the animal spirits made their way through the winding furrows of the cerebral cortex producing complex thoughts and behavioral responses such as anguish from the pain. Animal spirits transported in the nerves to the muscles did not inflate the muscles as proposed by Descartes but rather triggered a chemical reaction "a type of explosion" that caused the muscle to contract. Willis was an alchemist in addition to being a physician. In his book "Cerebri anatome" or

"The Anatomy of the Brain" published in 1664 Willis introduced the term "neurologie" to describe his "doctrine of the nerves".

The idea that pain was not a primary sensation but rather an emotion like pleasure dominated the thinking of physicians and philosophers from the time of Plato and Aristotle through the middle ages and even into modern times. Erasmus Darwin, a prominent English physician in the late eighteenth century and grandfather of Charles Darwin, argued that pain was not a special sense since it could be caused by extreme stimulation of any of the senses including light, sound, touch, hot and cold. The eighteenth century English philosopher David Hartley suggested that pain caused violent vibrations in the nerves and brain and that pain was pleasure carried beyond a due limit. The fact that pain lacked a specific sensory receptor such as those associated with vision, hearing, smell and taste no doubt influenced thinking that it was different from the primary senses.

Specific Nerves for Perception of Pain

Although the notion that separate nerves and separate pathways within the spinal cord and brain might exist for different sensations was entertained centuries before, coherent theories on how sensory nerves work did not develop until the nineteenth century. Nerves are formed at the spinal cord from two roots: a dorsal root at the back of the spinal cord and a ventral root at the front. Once they exit the bony spinal column through small openings in the bone called foramen, these nerves, spinal nerves, join together to form peripheral nerves (nerves away from the spinal cord) such as the sciatic nerve. A Scottish physician, Charles Bell, provided the first hint that the dorsal and ventral roots that form the spinal nerves had different functions when he needle pricked the ventral (front) root of an animal that had just died and observed contractions in muscles supplied by the nerve. When he pricked the dorsal (back) root there were no such contractions. He speculated that the ventral root carried motor signals from the brain to the muscles while the dorsal root likely provided nutrition for the nerve. Bell's observation stimulated the French physiologist François Magendie to perform a series of experiments on puppies in which he selectively cut the dorsal and ventral roots and then tested sensation and muscle function after they recovered from surgery. He found that the animals lost muscle function in the territory supplied by the cut ventral roots and lost sensory function including pain sensation in the territories supplied by the cut dorsal roots. Rather than a nutritional role as proposed by Bell, Magendie proved that the posterior roots carry sensory signals (touch, temperature and pain) from the peripheral nerves to the brain. His work on puppies set off a backlash regarding animal experimentation ultimately leading to the development of a major antivivisectionist movement in Europe.

In the mid nineteenth century, the English physician Augustus V. Waller conducted experiments in which he cut the dorsal sensory spinal roots in frogs and observed the effect on the nerve fibers on each side of the cut. There is a ganglion (group of nerve cell bodies) attached to the dorsal root, the dorsal root ganglion

(DRG) just before the two roots join together to form a spinal nerve (Fig. 2.2a). When Waller cut the dorsal root proximal (on the spinal cord side) to the DRG, the proximal root degenerated, on the other hand, if he cut the dorsal root distal (on the side away from the spinal cord) to the DRG the distal nerve fiber degenerated (Fig. 2.2b, c). He concluded that the DRG contained nerve cells that gave rise to two nerve fibers, one entering the spinal cord through the dorsal root and the other entering the spinal nerve. Even more important, he surmised that nerve cells must exert a trophic influence on their nerve fibers since cutting a nerve fiber leads to degeneration of the segment away from the nerve cell body. This conclusion, which is a fundamental principle of neuroscience, was remarkable given the fact that at the time it was not clear what the relationship was between the nerve cell bodies and nerve fibers. Subsequently, the process of degeneration of a nerve fiber after it is cut from its nerve cell body became know as Wallerian degeneration. As Waller predicted it provided a valuable tool that could be used to track the pathways of nerve fibers in the spinal cord and brain. One simply followed the degenerating nerve fibers under a microscope to see where they terminated.

Like many of his contemporaries, Waller had a wide range of scientific interests from the study of the molecular composition of clouds and fog in London to the study of the cellular mechanisms of inflammation. In 1861 he froze his own ulnar nerve at the elbow (using a combination of ice and salt for about an hour) and studied the effect on sensation and muscle control in his forearm and hand. The ulnar nerve is very close to the skin surface at the elbow (the "funny bone") which explains

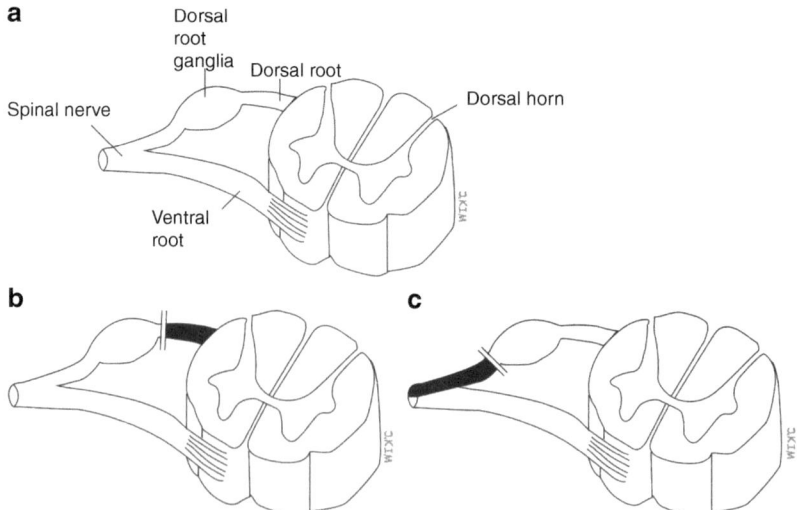

Fig. 2.2 Drawings illustrating Waller's experiment on cutting the sensory nerve root on each side of the dorsal root ganglia (DRG). (**a**) Spinal nerves are formed from a dorsal sensory root with the attached DRG and a ventral motor root. (**b**) If the dorsal root is cut proximal to the DRG, the proximal nerve fibers degenerate. (**c**) If the dorsal root is cut distal to the DRG, the distal nerve fibers degenerate

why it was easy for Waller to freeze the nerve and why you may get a sudden shock like sensation into your forearm and hand if you bump your elbow. Waller developed a complete loss of pain and touch sensation in the fourth and fifth fingers and the outside of the forearm and hand in the distribution of the ulnar nerve that lasted 10 days and he had a gradual return first of touch and then pain sensation over 5 months.

The pioneering German physiologist, Johannes Müller, was one of the first to suggest that there was specificity in the nerves sensing different sensations including pain. He pointed out that the type of sensation experienced by stimulating a nerve was largely determined by where the nerve fibers terminated in the brain. Müller's most famous pupil, Herman von Helmholz, divided the skin sensations into different modalities: touch, warm, cold and pain and suggested that these subsystems had the potential to interact with each other. This work was supported by the clinical observation that certain areas of the mucous membranes of the cheek and throat were sensitive to touch but not to pain while others were sensitive pain but not touch. By the end of the nineteenth century, anatomists had identified tiny nerve end organs in the skin thought to mediate the different types of sensation. The German physiologist, Max von Frey is credited with aligning the different end organs and free nerve endings in skin with the sensations of touch, warm, cold and pain. He felt that the nerves supplying each type of end organ went to specific areas of the brain. After assigning each end organ to a specific sensation (touch, warm, cold) the only unassigned nerve endings were the free nerve endings (unassociated with any sense organ) so he assigned them to pain. Furthermore, free nerve endings were by far most abundant consistent with the ubiquitous nature of pain. Further evidence for separation of sensory nerve functions came from experiments blocking peripheral nerves with freezing or compression such as performed by Waller. As the nerve was blocked cold and touch were the first sensations to go, followed by heat, superficial pain and finally by deep pain. With recovery of nerve function, the sensations returned in the reverse order.

As microscopes improved and better staining techniques were discovered, anatomists in the nineteenth century were able to study the microstructure of tissue for the first time. Nerve cells (called neurons) had two different kinds of branching processes: small tree like branches called dendrites and a long fiber that could extend for meters called an axon. Another pupil of Johannes Müller, Theodor Schwann, noted that the myelin that covers axons and gives them a glistening white appearance was generated by another cell separate from the neuron, now called a Schwann cell (Fig. 2.3). Each Schwann cell covers a segment of multiple axons with small gaps in between where one Schwann cell ends and the other starts. Schwann originally thought that the Schwann cells secreted the sheath called myelin but modern electron microscopy has shown that the multilayered sheath is composed of a folding of the Schwann cell membrane wrapped around the axon. Myelin acts as an insulator for the nerve fiber increasing the speed of conduction. Most sensory nerve axons have myelin sheaths but only about 20% of pain axons have myelin; the rest do not have myelin, the slowest conducting nerve fibers.

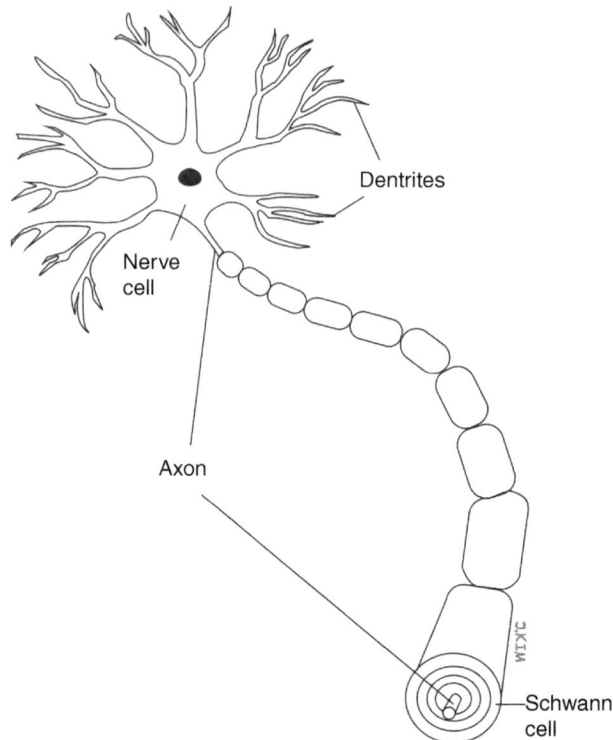

Fig. 2.3 Drawing of a nerve cell with its dendrites and single axon surrounded by myelin. The Schwann cells wrap themself around the axon to create the myelin sheath

A curious phenomenon first noted in the late nineteenth century was that a painful stimulus typically triggers a brief sharp stabbing pain followed a second or so later by a longer lasting burning pain. Various explanations for the phenomenon were suggested including stimulation of two different types of nerve endings or stimulation of nerve endings in different layers of the skin. Interestingly, the "first" pain is highly localized and well tolerated while the "second" pain is poorly localized and very poorly tolerated. We now know that these two different pain sensations are explained by two groups of nerve fibers with different speeds of conduction projecting to different areas of the brain.

How Do Free Nerve Endings of Pain Fibers Detect Noxious Stimuli?

Noxious stimuli are detected by a subpopulation of peripheral nerve fibers called pain fibers or nociceptors. The nerve cell bodies for these nerve fibers are located in the dorsal root ganglia (DRG) just outside of the spinal cord and their axons bifurcate and send one branch out to the periphery to detect the noxious stimuli and the other branch into the dorsal horn of the spinal cord to contact transmission neurons and interneurons that modify the signal on its way to the brain (see Fig. 2.2). Unlike other neurons in the brain that have dendrites to receive incoming signals and a single axon to transmit the signals to other neurons, the bifurcating axons of peripheral pain neurons can send and receive signals from either end. Not only does the central terminal release transmitters to activate target neurons, peripheral terminals release a variety of molecules that influence the area around the free nerve endings. For example, release of substance P causes dilation of blood vessels and an influx of inflammatory proteins from the blood.

As suggested earlier, pain fibers do not have specialized organs at their terminals for sensing noxious stimuli. Rather, their free nerve endings express a wide variety of membrane receptors that detect noxious stimuli (mechanical, thermal and chemical) and inflammatory factors. These receptors on the pain nerve endings have binding sites that recognize a specific molecule that in turn either opens ion channels causing the nerve fiber to fire or activate a second messenger inside the nerve terminal that can be transported back to the neuronal cell body where it can trigger new protein production. In a way, each of these tiny receptors represents a microscopic specialized end organ.

Peripheral pain neurons can be divided into multiple subsets based on the substances they release and the receptors expressed in their free nerve endings. The most common membrane receptors are a family of ion channel receptors, called TRPs for transient receptor potentials. TRPV1 is highly sensitive to heat and the chemical capsaicin found in chili peppers and is expressed in the majority of heat sensitive pain fiber endings. This explains why chili peppers cause a hot burning sensation when eaten and capsaicin in liniments causes burning pain when placed on the skin (see Liniments, Chap. 4). Other members of the receptor family have different mechanical and thermal sensitivities and respond to a variety of chemicals, for example cold sensitive receptors in pain fiber endings that also respond to menthol. This explains why a menthol lozenge produces a cool sensation in the mouth. Even though pain fibers have "free" nerve endings, each nerve ending has hundreds of molecular transducers (receptors) that sense specific noxious stimuli and chemicals.

With acute tissue injury not only do the pain axon terminals release neuropeptides that trigger inflammation but a variety of inflammatory cell types exit the blood and infiltrate the injured area. These cells in turn release a wide array of signaling molecules. The combination of the endogenous factors released by the pain nerve terminals and the inflammatory cells has been called "inflammatory soup". Remarkably, the free nerve endings of pain fibers express membrane receptors capable of recognizing and responding to hundreds of molecules in the inflammatory soup. Activation of these receptors increases the excitability of the pain fibers heightening their sensitivity to noxious stimuli. This explains why inflamed tissue is hypersensitive to pain. As we will see in Chap. 4, many commonly used pain medications such as aspirin and ibuprofen work at least in part by inhibiting enzymes (Cox-1 and Cox-2) that initiate synthesis of prostaglandins, an important component of inflammatory soup.

Pain Fibers in Nerve Sheaths (Nervi Nervorum)

In 1883, an English surgeon John Marshall, then president of the Royal College of Surgeons, speculated that the nerve sheath of peripheral nerves contained tiny nerves for sensing pressure and pain (nervi nervorum) just as other organs such as teeth and joints had such nerve terminals. He further speculated that certain anatomical locations such as the sciatic nerve in the pelvis were rich in these nerves. Marshall suggested that inflammation might result in the release of irritating materials and fluids (inflammatory soup) that excite the nervi nervorum and cause pain after nerve injury. He noted that tiny nerve fibers had been seen in the sheaths of nerves to the eye muscles but not in regular peripheral nerves and suggested that they should be looked for. A young surgical registrar working with Marshall, Victor Horsley, took up the challenge. He studied the peripheral nerves of human cadavers and identified small nerve fibers in the walls of the peripheral nerves (nervi nervorum) that were branches of the peripheral nerve, running first at right angles and then parallel to the nerve. Horsley felt that the nervi nervorum could explain sensitivity of peripheral nerves to stretch and pressure and also pain after nerve injury. Keep in mind that the nature of pain nerve endings was still being worked out at the time. Horsley's work was never published in full but only in abstract and 75 years passed before a Czech anatomist, Jan Hromada, confirmed Horsley's findings (even though he was unaware of them) and described free nerve ending in the sheaths of peripheral nerves. Pain fibers in the sheaths of peripheral nerves (nervi nervorum) are sensitive to the same mechanical, thermal, and chemical substances as pain fibers in other tissues.

Nerve Regeneration

With severe nerve damage, Wallerian degeneration occurs in the distal nerve fiber to create a favorable environment for new innervation. The release of growth factors by the injured nerves can lead to increased activity of ion channels in nearby uninjured nerve cells. Regenerating nerve fibers attempt to make their way back to the same tissue area they originally innervated. In order for this to occur, the Schwann cells that surrounded the damaged nerve fibers must remain intact. After transection of the axons, Schwann cells join together and form a tube that directs the regenerating axons to the right peripheral location. The Schwann cells also release growth factors that stimulate regrowth of the axon. If the Schwann cells are damaged and not available to direct the regenerating nerve, the sprouting axons may form a ball of growing axons, called a neuroma, at the nerve stump. Neuromas are sensitive to a range of chemicals, are extremely painful and can be relatively resistant to drug treatment.

Brain Pain Pathways

It wasn't until the mid nineteenth century that the spinal pathways for pain perception began to be clarified. Prior to that time all sensory signals to the brain were thought to travel uncrossed in the dorsal columns at the back of the spinal cord. In 1849, the French neurologist, Charles Edouard Brown-Séquard, observed that cutting the right half of the spinal cord in guinea pigs caused a loss of muscle function in the right leg and loss of pain sensation in the left leg. He concluded that the pain signals crossed after entering the spinal cord and ran up to the brain on the opposite side. A decade later he described detailed studies on patients with spinal cord damage where he precisely mapped the loss of sensation to pain, warmth, cold and touch and argued that each sensation ascended in different tracts in the spinal cord. The neurological sign of weakness in one leg and loss of pain and temperature sensation in the opposite leg (the Brown-Séquard sign) is still a reliable indicator of damage to half of the spinal cord (on the side of the weakness).

Brown-Séquard taught at Harvard Medical school and practiced neurology in New York and London before returning to Paris to succeed Claude Bernard as Professor of Experimental Medicine at the College of France. At the time, although Paris was the mecca of scientific medicine there was a wide chasm between advances in medical science and the routine practice of neurology. Brown-Séquard was considered at the forefront of scientific neurology yet his clinical practice still reflected ancient traditions. When the American abolitionist senator Charles Sumner visited Paris to recuperate from chronic pain due to injuries he had suffered in the Senate from a beating by the Southern congressman Preston Brooks, Sumner sought out the world renowned Brown-Séquard for a neurological consultation. Brown-Séquard spent 3 h examining Sumner in his hotel room and concluded that the beating had damaged several areas of Sumner's spinal cord and he recommended burning the skin over these areas with cotton soaked in a combustible substance (an ancient Japanese treatment called moxa or moxibustion). Sumner received six treatments from Brown-Séquard over 2 weeks. The pain was so intense that in the first session Sumner broke the chair he was gripping. Sumner suffered severe burns with the treatments and it took months for him to recuperate. Even though many friends and physicians in America were appalled at what they considered a reckless treatment, Summer later wrote to his friend Henry Longfellow that without this cruel treatment he might have become an invalid as Brown-Séquard warned.

By the mid twentieth century based on the work of neurologists and basic researchers an organized picture of spinal somatosensory transmission developed. Each sensory modality (e.g. pain, temperature, touch, and joint position sense) has unique nerves and nerve endings and the central axon of these nerves contacted distinct groups of transmission neurons in the spinal cord. Each group of transmission neurons in turn sends their axons in distinct bundles (tracts) up the spinal cord to different neuronal groups in the brain. They also send axon collaterals to interneurons and motor cells in the spinal cord.

However, as new technologies developed in the late twentieth century and it became possible to record from individual transmission neurons in the dorsal horn, a refined picture emerged. Nearly all transmission neurons in the dorsal horn of the spinal cord receive multiple sensory input signals and some receive signals from all sensory modalities. Researchers could find only a tiny subset of transmission neurons in the most superficial layer of the dorsal horn that received only pain signals. Therefore axons of most transmission neurons carry a convergence of sensory signals to the brain and the notion of individual sensory tracts is an oversimplification. These findings are not so surprising considering that a similar convergence of sensory signals is found in recordings from secondary neurons of other sensory modalities including hearing and vision. Convergence of sensory signals at the secondary neuronal level appears to be a basic principle of brain function. On the other hand, the fact that most transmission neuron axons carry a convergence of sensory signals does not mean that the pain signals are lost or that they cannot be reassembled and deciphered in different brain centers.

A number of secondary pain axons terminate in the lower brainstem upon a loosely organized group of neurons called the reticular formation. These connections are important for general arousal, activating brainstem reflexes resulting in hyperventilation, slowing of the heart rate and nausea. Another group of secondary pain axons terminate in two key areas of the brainstem, the rostroventralmedial region (RVM) of the medulla and the periaqueductal grey region (PAG) in the midbrain (Fig. 2.4). Neurons in the RVM and PAG send axons back down the spinal cord to activate interneurons in the dorsal horn that directly inhibit pain transmission completing a feedback loop. This inhibitory feedback system called the descending pain modulatory system (DPMS) is dependent on endogenous opioids and is a major reason for the analgesic effects of opioid drugs (see Chap. 7). The majority of secondary pain axons terminate in the thalamus, a nuclear structure deep in the center of the brain. The thalamus is a major relay center for all sensory signals arriving at the brain with different parts receiving different combinations of sensory inputs and projecting to different areas of the cortex. This segregation of sensory pathways into different brain regions is how the brain "knows" where the signal came from and what it means.

How Does the Brain Perceive Pain?

From an evolutionary point of view the sensation of pain is basic to all living organisms. Without the sensation of pain organisms lack the ability to respond to threats from the environment and would thus be easy prey to predators. Even the most primitive animals without a central brain have nerve ganglia containing nerve cells that receive pain signals and generate reflexive motor responses. As one moves out the evolutionary tree more complex brain structures evolve with higher and higher levels of complexity. Lower level reflexive behavior remains but under the control of the higher centers. For example, in humans, reflex withdraw from a painful stimulus occurs through neuronal networks in the spinal cord although these

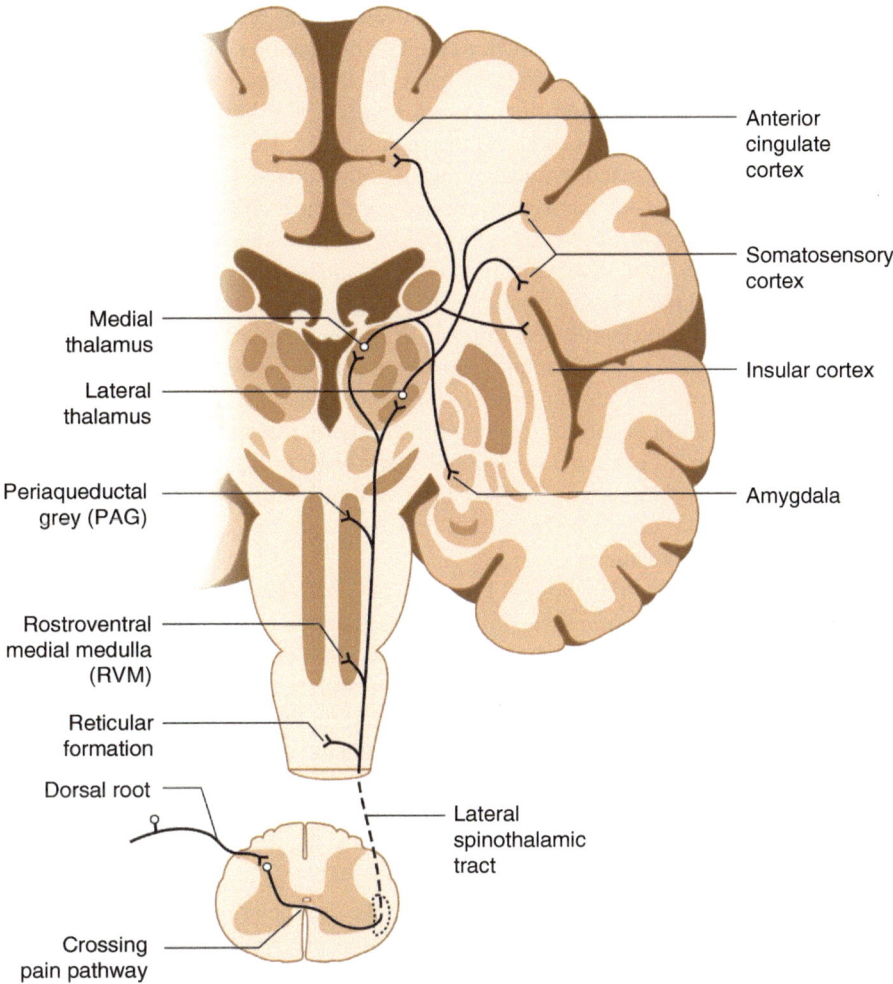

Fig. 2.4 Schematic drawing of spinal cord and brain pain pathways. *RF* reticular formation, *RVM* rostroventralmedial medulla, *PAG* periaqueductal grey

"automatic" reflexes can be modulated by higher brain levels. Since pain is closely associated with primitive reactions such as body postures, grimacing and "knitting" of the brow these "reflex" like behaviors are ingrained into more primitive levels of the evolving brain. In his book *The Expression of Emotions in Man and Animals* (1872) Charles Darwin suggested that these types of facial expressions were generated by predetermined nerve cell connections like a "habit". He studied the facial expressions of infants including keeping a daily log on the development of his own son and concluded that expressions such as crying and frowning were reflex actions reinforced by habit and did not imply awareness of pain. Although these reflex facial expressions were "hard wired" in the primitive brain he felt that a certain amount of practice was needed for full expression.

The concept of an evolutionary primitive "emotional brain" underlying a more advanced "thinking brain" dates back to the late nineteenth century and the famous English neurologist John Hughlings Jackson. Jackson, who was greatly influenced by Darwin, felt that evolution of the brain involved the build up of increasingly complex structures on top of more primitive structures. Jackson theorized that diseases like dementia caused symptoms by releasing lower primitive centers from higher control. Such a release from higher center control could make the most civilized man act like his primitive ancestors, a kind of reverse evolution. Jackson who was apprenticed to local physicians in York, England at the age of 15 had no formal university training but would go on to have a great influence on the developing field of Neurology. He is probably best known for his description of the slow march of muscle jerking along an extremity during a focal motor epileptic seizure, a "Jacksonian seizure". From this observation he surmised that there must be a topographical localization of different parts of the body on the motor cortex in the frontal lobe. Sigmund Freud acknowledged Jackson's profound influence on his psychoanalytic theory. The id was the primitive brain with raw passions and drives and the ego was the cognitive brain that prevented these passions and drives from breaking into consciousness.

In 1878, the French Neurologist, Paul Broca, who is best known for his work on localizing language function to the left frontal cortex, first used the term limbic lobe (from the Latin word for border, *limbus*) to describe a large arc of the medial cerebral cortex primarily composed of the cingulate and hippocampal cortex. In 1937, the American neurologist James Papez speculated on the role of the limbic lobe in emotion in a paper entitled "A proposed mechanism of emotion". He felt that the hypothalamus, the medial thalamic nucleus, and the cingulate and hippocampal cortex and their interconnections were key for feeling emotions and for emotional expression. American psychiatrist, Paul MacLean, coined the term "limbic system" to describe Papez's neural substrate for emotion. MacLean proposed an evolutionary based "triune brain theory" suggesting that the human brain is actually made up of three brains: the reptilian complex, the limbic system (paleomammalian) and the neocortex (neomamallian). The basic idea is that during vertebrate brain evolution there are periods of stability followed by bursts of expansion resulting in these three main layers of hierarchy. The reptilian or "R" brain is concerned with instinctual primitive survival functions such as exploration, feeding, and aggression. The limbic system is the emotional brain that generates fear, anger and sexual behavior and controls the emotional response to incoming signals such as pain and pleasure. Finally, the neocortex is the highest level of cognitive functioning involved in, abstraction, planning and reasoning.

Although MacLean's triune model is clearly an oversimplification of brain evolution and comparative anatomy it does serve as a useful didactic model for understanding how the brain perceives pain. Central pain pathways can be divided into three systems roughly corresponding to the triune model. The most primitive system, the spinal cord, brainstem and basal ganglia results in reflexive instinctual responses from simple withdraw of an extremity to behavioral responses such as facial grimacing and pacing. The intermediate system, the limbic system, generates emotions such as fear and anger and controls the emotional response. Finally, the highest system, the neocortex generates the discriminatory component of pain perception. This system provides declarative knowledge about the world based on the combined input from all the senses. In summary we perceive pain at multiple levels: a purely instinctual level, an emotional level and a knowledge level.

Pain as an Emotion

In the mid-twentieth century as our understanding of the molecular mechanisms of pain transmission within the brain expanded pain researchers emphasized the dual nature of pain. Even though there clearly is a sensory component to pain with sensory receptors that feed into central sensory discriminative centers they emphasized that there also is a psychological component that is highly individual and influenced by past experience. The pendulum even began to swing back toward the notion that pain wasn't a primary sensation at all but rather an emotion. In an article "On the nature of Pain" published in the journal *Brain* in 1957, the English neurologist William Gooddy emphasized that although impulse patterns in nerves and nerve centers may provide the neurophysiological basis for pain and may influence the quality of pain, they did not determine whether or not an individual experiences pain.

In his article entitled "Psychogenic pain and pain-prone patients" published in the *American Journal of Medicine* in 1959, University of Rochester Psychiatrist George Engel emphasized that pain is both a sensation and a personal experience that others can't appreciate. What an individual experiences during painful stimuli is a complex psychological phenomenon and is not always unpleasant. As one of many examples he noted that at the height of sexual excitement some people enjoy pain. This can become the dominant feature of sexual activity leading to sadomasochism. He also emphasized that in "pain prone patients" psychic factors can play a primary role in the genesis of pain even in the absence of peripheral afferent stimulation.

At the turn of the twenty-first century Bud Craig, a pain researcher at the Barrow Neurological Institute in Phoenix Arizona suggested that pain is a homeostatic emotion. He defined homeostasis as a dynamic and ongoing process with the goal of maintaining an optimal balance in the physiological condition of the body. He likened pain to other homeostatic mechanisms such as temperature control, itch, hunger and thirst control. Each of these systems has sensory monitors along with reflex and behavioral responses to maintain homeostasis. For example, all mammals regulate body temperature by monitoring core and skin temperature and adjusting autonomic (cardiorespiratory) activity to change blood flow to the body core and skin while at the same time altering behavior by leaving a hot or cold area or in the case of humans adding or subtracting clothes. In primates, a forebrain system evolved that contains an afferent representation of the physiological condition of the body the so-called "feeling self".

Although pain awareness occurs at multiple levels within the central nervous system perception and insight into the meaning of pain require higher cortical function. But what areas of the cerebral cortex are necessary? The problem is analogous to asking what areas are necessary for consciousness. We don't really know but likely multiple interconnecting nerve centers are involved. Stimulation of the medial thalamus that projects to the insular cortex and other parts of the limbic system in patients undergoing surgery for implantation of deep brain stimulators can reproduce pain sensations experienced earlier in life including the emotional content of the pain. The limbic system including the insular cortex along with the mesial temporal lobe structures, the amygdala and hippocampus appear to be critical for pain memory as well as emotion. Damage to these areas in patients can impair emotional and motivational responses to painful stimuli. By comparison the lateral thalamus projects to the parietal and frontal lobes areas critical for cognitive assessment of the pain and assessment of the future consequences of pain. Damage to these pathways typically does not cause pain or alter the perception of pain but it does alter how we react to pain.

Suggested Additional Reading

Craig AD. A new view of pain as a homeostatic emotion. Trends Neurosci. 2003;26:303–7.

Darwin C. The expression of the emotions in man and animals. London: John Murray; 1872.

Maclean PD. The triune brain in evolution: role in paleocerebral function. New York: Plenum Press; 1990.

Papez JW. A proposed mechanism of emotion. Arch Neurol Psychiatr. 1937;38:725–43.

Rey R. The history of pain. Trans. By Wallace LE, Cadden JA, Cadden SW. London: Harvard University Press; 1995.

Chapter 3
What Causes Sciatica?

Most ancient people thought that painful diseases like sciatica resulted from evil spirits that invaded the body through the "sinister" left nostril or left ear producing pain by infiltrating the blood vessels and heart. Of the many Egyptian gods Sekhmet and Seth were most commonly associated sciatica. The sudden violent sharp pain of sciatica was called the witch's shot in Germany and in England, the elf's arrow. Around the fifth century B.C., Hippocrates and his fellow Greek physicians challenged the notion that diseases resulted from supernatural forces. Hippocrates felt that sciatica resulted from damage to the hip. He observed that it was particularly common during summer and autumn and he speculated that hot weather led to drying up of the joint fluid. From what we know today, this seasonal occurrence was probably due to injuries from increased physical activities such as farming and athletic events common at that time of the year.

As the Greek Empire began to crumble and to be replaced by the Roman Empire many prominent Greek physicians moved to Rome to practice medicine and serve the wealthy Roman landlords. The best-known physician of the Roman Empire was Galen who was born in the Greek city of Pergamon in 130 A.D. and received his medical training in Alexandria. He lived most of his life in Rome where he was court physician to four successive emperors. Like Hippocrates, Galen associated sciatica with hip disease and attributed sciatica to a range of disorders including dislocation of the hip, bony tuberculosis, gout and even polio. Like most others at the time he did not differentiate between pain arising from the hip joint or spine. Galen recognized several types of pain based on the quality (throbbing, heavy, stretching, lancinating) and felt that the patient's description of pain could help with the diagnosis. For example, throbbing pain suggested an inflammation whereas a heavy and stretching pain suggested a tumor. Galen dissected a range of animals but not humans and his understanding of the spine and nerves was dominated by his belief in animal spirits and body humors. He treated sciatica with blood letting to release the toxic humors.

The best early clinical description of sciatica was provided by the Roman physician, Caelius Aurelianus, in the fourth century AD. A severe pain began in the lower back and radiated into the buttock, calf, foot and toes. The pain could be accompa-

© Springer International Publishing AG, part of Springer Nature 2019
R. W. Baloh, *Sciatica and Chronic Pain*,
https://doi.org/10.1007/978-3-319-93904-9_3

nied by low-back spasms, loss of sensation and even muscle wasting in the leg in chronic cases. Aurelianus noted that straining with bowel movement could cause a shooting pain into the toes and that some patients developed a crooked posture and inability to bend forward. Further he suggested that a sudden jerk during exercise, lifting a heavy object from a low place, excessive digging in the ground, a bad fall and excessive sexual activity could cause sciatica. Like most others at the time he did not differentiate between pain arising from the hip joint or spine.

As with most other areas of medicine there was little progress in understanding of the vertebral column, spine and nerves over the next ten centuries. In 1543, Andreas Vesalius, the first in a long line of great anatomists to study and work at the University of Padua in Italy, published his monumental De Humani Corporis Fabrica (On the fabric of the human body) that for the first time provided a comprehensive description of the human body with 273 illustrations. Although human autopsies had been performed many times in prior centuries Vesalius was the first to systematically document his extensive experience with human dissections. To give some idea of how ingrained Galen's teachings on anatomy were within the medical community, a well known physician at the time of Vesalius, Jacques du Bois of Amiens, remarked that any structure found in contemporary man that differed from Galen's description could only be due to a "decadence and degeneration in mankind". Vesalius described the vertebral column and the spinal nerves and clearly distinguished between nerves, tendons and ligaments. He emphasized that nerves originate from the brain and spinal cord and were not hollow effectively debunking the long held theory of Galen and Decartes that nerves were tubes for conducting fluid from the ventricles (known as *succus nerveus,* nerve juice at the time of Vesalius).

A major breakthrough in understanding of sciatica came in the mid eighteenth century when the Italian anatomist and physician, Domenico Cotugno, differentiated sciatic nerve pain from hip pain. Cutugno is probably best known for discovery of cerebrospinal fluid, the fluid bathing the brain and spinal canal. He dissected cadavers while they were standing to demonstrate circulation of spinal fluid between the brain and spinal column. He surmised that spinal fluid was formed by exudation from small arteries in the dura and resorbed by small veins. Cutugno noted that the nerve roots leaving the spine had dural sleeves filled with spinal fluid and he speculated that acrid matter accumulated in the sheaths of the spinal nerves that form the sciatic nerve causing pain and weakness along its course. For more than a century sciatica became known as Cotugno's syndrome.

Cotugno was a remarkable man with many accomplishments who came from humble origins to become professor of anatomy and surgery at the Neapolitan hospital and royal physician to the king of Naples. He was a Latin scholar and humanist who was an expert in art, architecture and antiquities. He is not only known for his work on spinal fluid and sciatica but he was a pioneer in the study of the inner ear and was the first to describe the fluids in the inner ear.

Although early physicians recognized that back pain and sciatica were commonly associated with heavy labor and trauma the mechanism of that association was unknown. In the mid-nineteenth century, the famous Viennese pathologist, Carl Rokitansky, first noted forward displacement of the fifth lumbar vertebral body at autopsy due to fracture of the bony lamina stabilizing the back of the vertebral column. The condition became know as spondylolisthesis from the Greek words spóndylos meaning vertebra (back bone) and listhesis, displacement. Clinical descriptions of patients who developed sciatica due to spondylolisthesis during pregnancy and after trauma soon followed. One of the first cases reported in the United States was a young woman who gained 100 lb during her pregnancy. The increased weight led to a stress fracture of bone stabilizing the spine. A controversy arose as to whether the fracture and the associated displacement of the vertebral body resulted from chronic stress on a normal bone or from an underlying developmental bony defect. By the early twentieth century most agreed that spondylolisthesis usually results from a stress fracture of normal bone. This concept was consistent with the finding of a high incidence of these spinal abnormalities in military recruits carrying heavy backpacks and in young athletes particularly gymnasts. Interestingly, stress fractures of the spine have been identified in skeletal remains dating back as far as 6000 BC and the condition appears to be exclusive to primates who stand and walk upright.

Prior to the twentieth century, clinicians lumped back pain and sciatica together as lumbago, a type of rheumatism of the low back. The word rheumatism comes from the Greek word rheumatismos that means to suffer from a flux or flow. Although scientific medicine was beginning to influence thinking in the medical community in the nineteenth century, archaic theories involving body humors and vital forces still dominated the routine clinical practice of medicine. In 1864, the French physician Ernest Lasègue described a simple bedside test to diagnose sciatica ("the straight leg raising test") in which he lifted the extended leg while the patient lay supine. Patients with sciatica would develop severe pain in the affected extremity due to stretching of the spinal nerve that was being compressed.

The current concept that sciatica commonly results from an irritation of one of the spinal nerves that form the sciatic nerve from injury or degeneration of the spine began to develop at the turn of the twentieth century. In a key paper published in the English journal *Lancet* in 1927, an Italian orthopedic surgeon, Vittorio Putti, pointed out that arthritic degenerative disease (osteoarthritis) of the lumbar intervertebral foramen, the bony canals through which spinal nerves exit the spine, was a common cause of sciatica. He went on to recommend conservative medical management of the arthritis but noted that if medical treatment wasn't effective surgical resection of the degenerating bone was possible.

A major breakthrough came in 1934 when William Mixter and Joseph Barr published their classic paper on herniated intervertebral discs in the New England Journal of Medicine. They convincingly showed that a ruptured disc could press on one of the lower lumbar or sacral spinal nerves as they exit the spinal canal producing typical sciatica. Furthermore, they showed that surgical removal of the offending protruded disc could cure the sciatica. Mixter was the chief of neurosurgery at the Massachusetts General Hospital (following in the footsteps of Harvey Cushing) and Barr was an orthopedic surgeon at the MGH. Since that time, the idea that disc herniation and bony degeneration are the most common causes of sciatica has dominated medical thinking. The big controversy, as we will see later, is how to manage these common spinal disorders.

Structure of the Spine and Sciatic Nerve

Before considering the causes of sciatica one must have a basic understanding of the anatomy of the spine and the sciatic nerve (Fig. 3.1). The reader will probably want to refer back to this figure from time to time when reading the remaining chapters. The spinal column is made up of four segments, cervical, thoracic, lumbar and sacral (Fig. 3.1a). Spinal nerves are formed at the spinal cord from two roots, a sensory root at the back and a motor root at the front (see Fig. 2.1). Pairs of spinal nerves exit the spine through bony canals on each side and are named for the

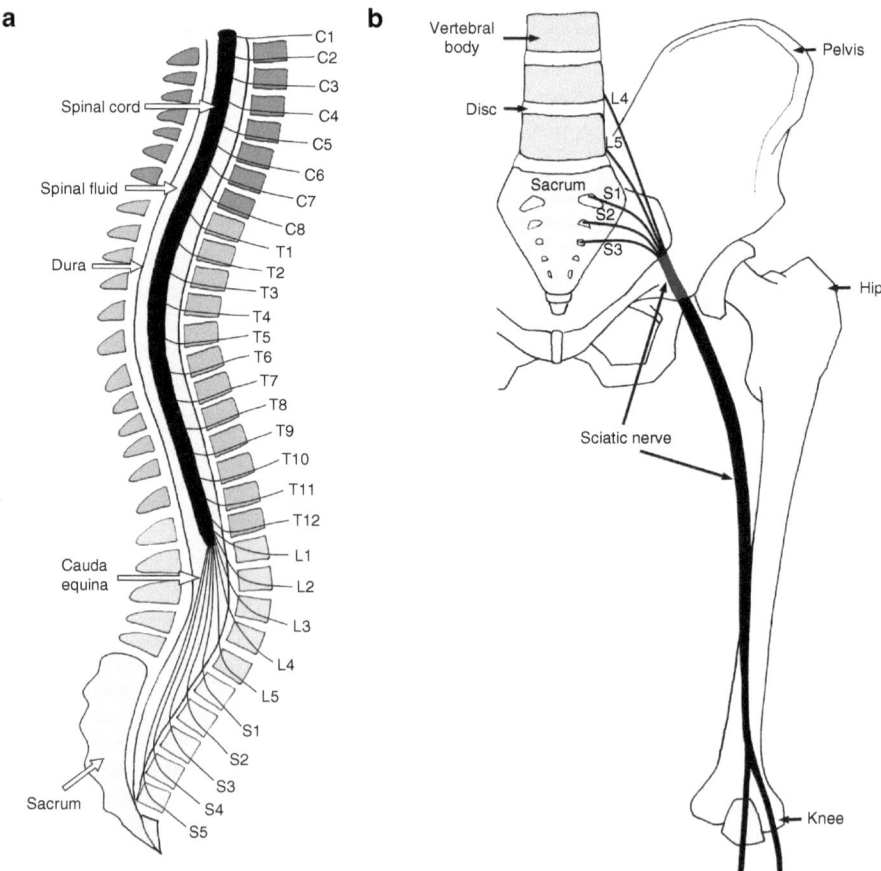

Fig. 3.1 Anatomy of the lumbosacral spine and sciatic nerve. (**a**) Lateral view of the lumbosacral spine showing the spinal cord and spinal nerves exiting the spine on the right side. Note that the spinal cord ends at the T12 level and all of the spinal nerves exit the cord at that level. (**b**) Formation of the sciatic nerve in the pelvis. After the L4, L5, S1, S2 and S3 spinal nerves exit the spine they join together to form the sciatic nerve. The sciatic nerve bifurcates just above the knee to form the peroneal and tibial nerves. C cervical, T thoracic, L lumbar, S sacral

vertebra directly above where they exit, for example spinal nerve L1 exits the spine below the first lumbar vertebra. The dura (also called the dura mater) is the thick fibrous membrane that together with the thin arachnoid membrane encloses the spinal fluid that surrounds the spinal cord and spinal nerves in the spinal canal. The spinal cord ends near the junction of the thoracic and lumbar spine so that all of the lumbar and sacral spinal nerves exit the spinal cord at that level. The collection of spinal nerves below the ending of the spinal cord is called the cauda equina (Latin for "horse's tail") because of the similarities in appearance to that of a horse's tail (Fig. 3.1a).

The fourth and fifth lumbar spinal nerves and the first three sacral spinal nerves leave their bony canal and join together to form the sciatic nerve in the pelvis (Fig. 3.1b). Sciatica can result from damage to the spinal nerves that form the sciatic nerve anywhere from the cauda equina to their joining together in the pelvis and from damage to the sciatic nerve anywhere before it divides above the knee. Damage to the spinal cord itself would invariably cause many other symptoms in addition to sciatica and damage to the branches of the sciatic nerve at the knee would cause pain in the lower leg not in the back, buttock and thigh.

Identifying the Cause of Sciatica

Traditionally neurologists are taught to first identify the anatomical site of a lesion (area of damage) based on the history and examination. Localization of the lesion requires knowledge of anatomy, in the case of sciatica the anatomy illustrated in Fig. 3.1. The skills needed to obtain the patient history and perform a neurological examination require years of training and are still part of the "art of medicine" but anyone can recognize the key features of sciatica – pain radiating down the leg into the foot usually without any other abnormalities. The list of causes of sciatica is long and will be addressed in more detail later in this chapter. I teach students to focus on the common causes with the old adage that if one hears hoof beats it is usually best to think of horses and not zebras. On the other hand, it is important to know that "zebras" exist and to at least be aware of rare causes. Here the concept of "red flags" comes in handy. These are symptoms or findings that suggest that something atypical and potentially more serious is going on and maybe one should think about "zebras" (Table 3.1).

Overview of the Common Causes of Sciatica

Spinal column disorders account for about 85% of all cases of sciatica. There are three major spinal column disorders that cause sciatica: (1) herniated discs, (2) osteoarthritis with bony overgrowth, and (3) displacement of a vertebra, spondylolisthesis. All three can compress spinal nerves in the cauda equina or in the bony

Table 3.1 Sciatica "Red Flags" that may require immediate action

Red flag	Possible diagnoses
Major trauma prior to onset	Vertebral bone fracture and displacement, traumatic nerve injury
Known cancer, particularly involving pelvic organs	Compression of nerves in the cauda equina or pelvis by metastasis or primary tumor
Known infection	Abscess with compression of spinal or sciatic nerves
Unremitting pain	Compression of nerves in the cauda equina or pelvis by metastasis or primary tumor
Worsening of pain at night when sleeping	Tumor of the cauda equine particularly a schwannoma
Pain in both legs when walking	Spinal stenosis
Weakness in one or both legs	Disk herniation, spinal stenosis, bone displacement, tumor of cauda equina
Bowel and bladder dysfunction	Midline disk herniation, spinal stenosis, bone displacement, tumor of cauda equina
Saddle anesthesia (numbness in a saddle distribution)	Midline disk herniation, spinal stenosis, bone displacement, tumor of cauda equina

canal as they exit the spine. As a rule herniated discs occur in middle age people (30–60 years), osteoarthritis in older people (>60 years) and spondylolisthesis occurs in younger people (<30 years). The remaining 15% of cases of sciatica have many causes. Spinal nerves can be compressed by tumors, cysts, infection and normal or abnormal blood vessels. The sciatic nerve can be entrapped and compressed within the pelvis by muscles or tendons, by tumors, or by bleeding after trauma. An enlarged uterus either due to pregnancy or later in life due to endometriosis is a frequent cause of sciatica in women. Sciatic neuritis (inflammation of the sciatic nerve) can occur in isolation or be part of a systemic viral infection.

Distinguishing Between Common Causes of Sciatica

The flow chart in Fig. 3.2 provides an overview for deciding on the likely cause of sciatica. Of the common causes herniated discs, spondylolisthesis and infection usually develop rapidly whereas osteoarthritis, tumors and nerve entrapment typically develop gradually. Sudden onset in a middle aged person after lifting, straining or vigorous exercise suggests a herniated disc while sudden onset in a young person after trauma or vigorous sport suggests vertebral displacement with spondylolisthesis. Infection of the sciatic nerve typically has a rapid onset (minutes to hours) and may be associated with the rash of herpes zoster (shingles) or systemic symptoms such as fever chills and malaise. Gradual onset of sciatica in an older person with a history of chronic back pain suggests osteoarthritis with foramen or spinal stenosis (narrowing). Gradual onset of pain that is continuous or slowly progressive and is aggravated by lying down suggests a tumor compressing a spinal nerve or the sciatic

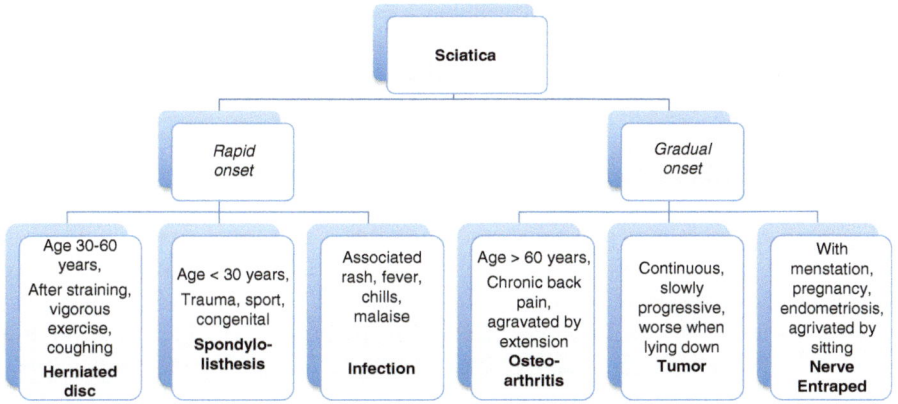

Fig. 3.2 Flow chart illustrating how to distinguish between the common causes of sciatica

nerve. Finally, gradual onset of sciatica associated with menstruation, pregnancy, or endometriosis and is aggravated by prolonged sitting suggests sciatic nerve entrapment.

Sciatica pain typically begins in the low back and radiates to the lower buttock and in a narrow band down the leg in different locations depending on which spinal nerve is involved (see Fig. 3.1). With L4 spinal nerve involvement the band radiates to the front of the thigh and can be confused with hip pain. With L5 spinal nerve involvement the band radiates down the outside of the thigh toward the front of the calf and into the great toe while with S1 spinal nerve involvement the pain radiates down the back of the thigh to the outside of the calf and into the outside of the foot. When the sciatic nerve is compressed in the pelvis the band of pain down the leg is much broader and often there is no associated back pain. Sciatica is usually just on one side since discs typically rupture to the side and arthritic bony overgrowth usually starts on one side but both sides can be involved if for example, a vertebra is displaced backward (spondylolisthesis), a disc herniates straight back or osteoarthritis narrows the entire spinal canal, so called spinal stenosis. Sciatica involving both legs brought on by walking (neurogenic claudication) suggests compression of the cauda equina usually associated with spinal stenosis.

Causes of Rapid Onset Sciatica

Herniated Discs

Each intervertebral disc contains a gelatinous center surrounded by a fibrous band, which in turn is surrounded by a strong ligament (Fig. 3.3a). The outer ligament is innervated with pain fibers but there is no innervation to the body of the disc. With trauma and aging, degenerative arthritic changes occur in the gelatinous center and the surrounding fibrous disc. The gelatinous center slowly loses water content and degrades from a resilient gel to a hardened substance. The discs tend to flatten resulting in increased pressure on the facet joints causing hypertrophy of the joints. Disc protrusions (where the gelatinous center bulges through the fibrous disc but is held in check by the annular ligament) occur in more than 50% of normal people, particularly in the low back region. Pain can result from activation of nerve endings in the outer ligament, compression of a spinal nerve, or an inflammatory response triggered by chemicals released from the bulging disc. An actual rupture of the gelatinous center through the outer ligament (Fig. 3.3b) is less common but even that can occur in normal subjects without symptoms of sciatica. Interestingly, disc often herniate in the morning not long after getting out of bed. Presumably, during the night, pressure on the intervertebral discs is decreased allowing rehydration of the gelatinous center. In the morning after getting up, there is a sudden increase in

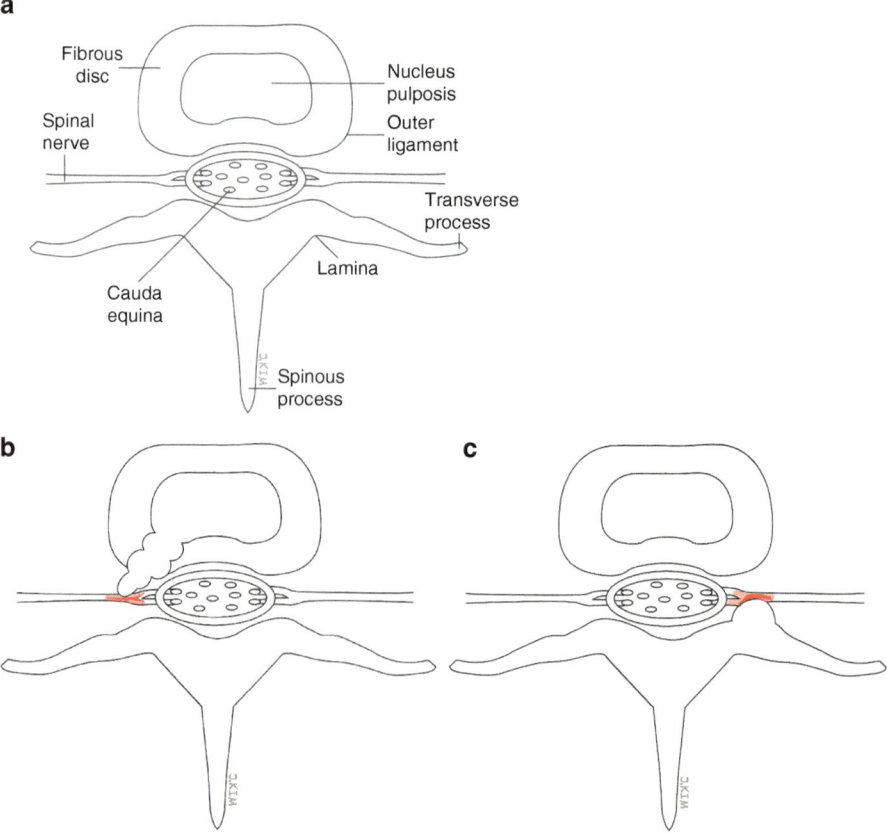

Fig. 3.3 Lumbosacral spinal nerve compression at the bony foramen. (**a**) Normal anatomy. (**b**) Herniated disc compressing the spinal nerve. (**c**) Bony overgrowth due to osteoarthritis compressing the spinal nerve

pressure on the discs due to the weight of the vertebral column. Vigorous early morning exercises, particularly weight lifting, could lead to a disc rupture as the vertical load on the disc exceeds the strength of the outer ligament.

Spondylolisthesis

As a rule fracture of a vertebral bone does not cause sciatica unless there is destabilization of the spinal column. It is a common cause of back pain, however, and fracture is a common cause of back pain in adolescent athletes. Fracture of the key stabilizing elements of the vertebra can lead to dislocation with forward displacement of the vertebral body and compression of spinal nerves causing sciatica (Fig. 3.4). Spondylolisthesis can result from trauma and developmental bony defects. Diseases involving the vertebra such as osteoporosis, Paget's disease, infections and cancer (primary and metastatic) can predispose to bony fractures and spinal column displacement. Severe osteoporosis can cause a sudden collapse of a vertebra.

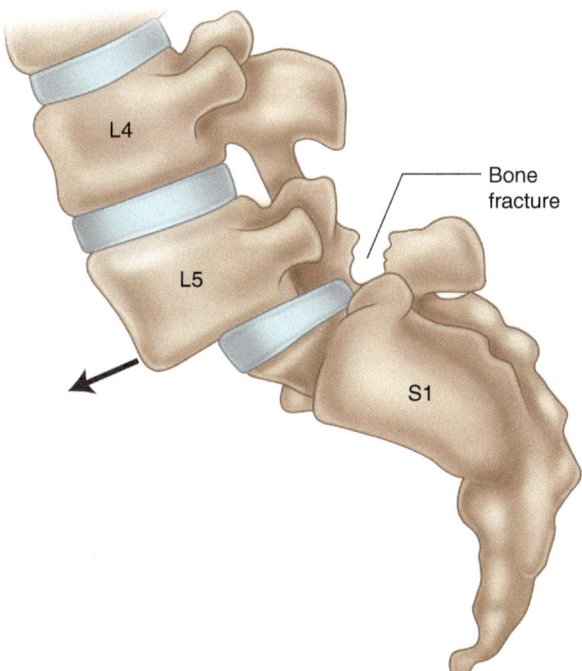

Fig. 3.4 Spondylolisthesis at the lumbosacral junction. Fracture of the stabilizing elements of the spine causes dislocation with forward movement of the L5 vertebral body on the S1 vertebral body

Infections

Infection involving the spine or the pelvis can cause sciatica by direct involvement of a nerve or by compression. Abscesses just outside the spine or in the pelvic organs can present with sciatica. Herpes zoster infection of the sciatic nerve (shingles) can mimic a disc herniation with the acute onset of severe sciatica without systemic symptoms of infection. The key to the diagnosis is to identify the typical vesicular rash on the skin that may be delayed for a few days after the onset of the leg pain.

Causes of Gradual Onset Sciatica

Osteoarthritis

This category best fits with the nonspecific terms lumbago and rheumatism used by eighteenth and nineteenth century physicians. Stated simply osteoarthritis represents degeneration of the spine due to a lifetime of wear and tare. With aging, degenerative arthritic changes not only occur in the discs but also in the vertebral joints, ligaments and surrounding bone. There is associated hypertrophy of the joint membranes and small synovial cysts (a fluid filled pouching of the synovial lining of the joint) are common. With the aging of the general population and the overall increased life span osteoarthritis has replaced herniated discs as the most common cause of sciatica. Foramen stenosis refers to a narrowing of the bony canal where the spinal nerves exit the spine (Fig. 3.3c) and spinal stenosis refers to narrowing of the entire spinal canal. Both conditions tend to be aggravated by bending backward and relieved by bending forward and lying down. Sciatica due to osteoarthritis is slower and more gradual in onset than that due to herniated discs but occasionally the pain can change suddenly, particularly if a synovial cyst develops and compresses the root exiting the narrowed foramen. Spinal stenosis leads to compression of the cauda equina and commonly causes pain with walking and multiple other neurological symptoms including leg weakness, numbness and impaired bowel and bladder function.

Tumors

Benign and malignant tumors can infiltrate or compress the spinal nerves anywhere from where they exit the spinal cord to where they come together to form the sciatic nerve or can involve the sciatic nerve itself in the pelvis prior to its branching in the leg (see Fig. 3.1). The most common benign tumor to cause sciatica is a schwannoma originating from the schwann cells that produce the insulation lining of nerves (see Fig. 2.2). These tumors can involve the spinal nerves of the cauda equina inside the spinal fluid space, at the intravertebral foramen after the nerves have exited the dura, or they can originate from the sciatic nerve in the pelvis. They often develop at the intervertebral foramen producing a "dumbbell" like shape with one head inside and the other outside the foramen. The genetic disorder neurofibromatosis type II (so-called NF2) is associated with multiple schwannomas throughout the body. A wide range of malignant tumors can produce sciatica with the most common being metastatic cancer from kidney, lung and breast and primary tumors of bone. Progressive sciatica can be the presenting symptom of an enlarging pelvic tumor such as a large ovarian cyst or ovarian and uterine cancer. Cyclical sciatica can be associated with endometriosis (a disorder where tissue that normally lines the uterus grows outside the uterus in the pelvis). In one survey, half of patients with endometriosis complained of intermittent pain radiating down one or both legs.

Nerve Entrapment

Pain due to nerve entrapment by normal tissue such as a muscle or ligament is not uncommon. A good example is the carpal tunnel syndrome where the median nerve is compressed at the wrist. Many women develop carpal tunnel syndrome during pregnancy due to swelling of the tissue at the wrist. As noted earlier in this chapter, sciatica is common late in pregnancy as the sciatic nerve is trapped between the fetal head and pelvic brim. Sciatica immediately after delivery can be due to stretching of the nerve by prolonged positioning with the legs in outward rotation, trauma from forceps or entrapment by injured muscles or tendons near the nerve. As wallets have become stuffed with credit cards there are reports of sciatica being relieved by removing a bulging wallet from the back pocket, so-called credit-carditis. Presumably other objects such as tools or golf balls in the back pocket or prolonged sitting on a hard surface can also cause or aggravate sciatica due to entrapment of the sciatic nerve.

After leaving the spine through their bony canals the lumbar and sacral spinal nerves enter the pelvis combining to form the sciatic nerve directly behind the piriformis muscle (Fig. 3.5). In at least one in ten people, part or all of the nerve actually penetrates the muscle. With the piriformis syndrome, the sciatic nerve is entrapped by muscle or surrounding tissue as the nerve passes by or through it. Whether the nerve is entrapped by a normal muscle or by a muscle that has been injured from running or lunging is often unclear but probably there are multiple different mechanisms for the entrapment. The typical symptom complex includes: pain in the mid-buttock, worsening of pain with outward rotation of the hip, tenderness at the back of the hip (in the so-called sciatic notch area), and worsening of pain with prolonged sitting. There are few conditions in medicine more controversial than the piriformis syndrome. Some think it is the most common cause of sciatica (including several sites on the internet) while others doubt it exists (including several of my neurological colleagues). As we will see in Chap. 5 newer imaging techniques can identify sciatic nerve compression by the piriformis muscle but so far only a few cases have been documented with these techniques.

Fig. 3.5 Relationship between the sciatic nerve and the piriformis muscle in the pelvis. In approximately 90% of individuals the sciatic nerve runs under the muscle as shown and in the remaining 10% of individuals all or part of the nerve penetrates the muscle

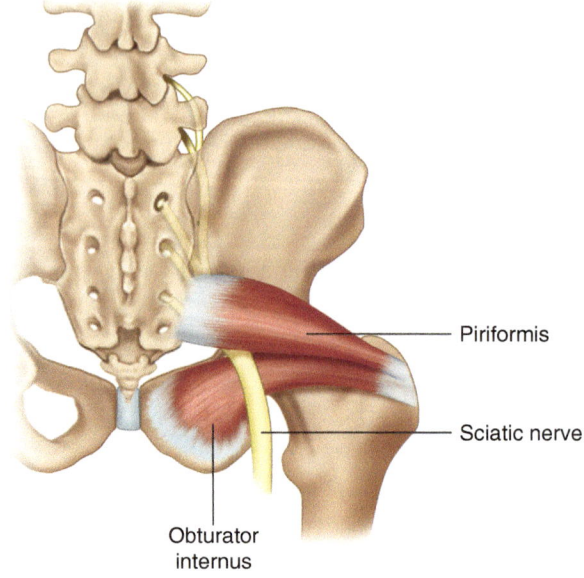

Piriformis

Sciatic nerve

Obturator
internus

Illustrative Cases

Case 1

Alfredo, a 45 years old gardener, suddenly developed excruciating pain radiating down his right leg. He had been lifting blocks to build a wall the day before the onset of the pain and had some back pain that night but he took ibuprofen and had a reasonably good night sleep. The next morning after getting out of bed and reaching down to put on his pants the pain hit him. Initially he could not move and he screamed for his wife to help him get down to the floor where he assumed a fetal position and refused to move. She gave him two ibuprofen tablets and after a few hours she helped him get into bed even though the movement caused severe pain. She called his primary care physician who suggested that he probably had sciatica and that he should take ibuprofen every 6 h and arrange an appointment to see her. Getting up to go to the bathroom resulted in excruciating pain and he could not put any weight on his painful leg. Fortunately his wife kept a set of crutches from a prior ankle injury and he found that with the crutches he could move about although he dreaded getting in and out of bed. In his doctor's office he complained of markedly worsened pain when his right leg was elevated while supine (a positive straight-leg-raising test) but otherwise his examination was normal without any weakness or loss of sensation in the right leg. He reported that the pain went down the outside of his leg into the great toe and pad of his foot.

Comment

Based on his age, the sudden onset of excruciating pain, and the positive straight-leg-raising test the most likely cause of Alfredo's pain was a herniated disc. The pain followed the sensory distribution of the right L5 spinal nerve so the disc between the L5 and S1 vertebra probably ruptured compressing the right L5 spinal nerve. There were no red flags.

Case 2

Lamar, a 20 years old college gymnast, complained of back pain after a fall when attempting a forward dismount on his parallel bars routine. The pain was just in the back for a few days but then it began shooting down the back of both legs into the foot. The pain improved when he leaned forward such as when walking upstairs but was worse when extending backward. He continued to attend classes but could not exercise without aggravating the pain. When examined by the team's sports physician he had a positive straight-leg-raising test on both sides and but otherwise his examination was normal.

Comment

Based on his age, rapid onset after trauma and involvement of both sides, the cause of Lamar's sciatica was most likely spondylolisthesis compressing multiple spinal nerves. He had a clear red flag, onset after trauma.

Case 3

In my case (a 62 years old man at the time) described briefly in the Preface, I had the gradual onset of right-sided pain that was slowly progressing. I had back pain but the most bothersome pain was a constant dull ache (like a toothache) in the back of the right buttock at times with a sharp pain radiating into the outside of my thigh and calf. The pain was worse after sitting for any length of time so I needed to frequently get up and walk or stand when in meetings or lectures. I had no numbness or weakness in the leg and my pain was only slightly increased with the straight-leg-raising test.

Comment

Based on the slow progression and my age at the time, the likely diagnosis was osteoarthritis with foramen stenosis compressing L5 on the right (focusing on the horses and not the zebras). At that time, there were no red flags.

Suggested Additional Reading

Mixter WJ, Barr JS. Rupture of the intervertebral disc with involvement of the spinal cord. N Engl J Med. 1934;211:210–4.
Ropper AH, Zafonte RD. Sciatica. N Engl J Med. 2015;372:1240–8.

Chapter 4
Initial Management of Sciatica

Since in early times sciatica was attributed to evil spirits, treatments such as chants, rituals and back manipulations were designed to force out the evil spirits. Hippocrates and his followers used moderate therapeutic interventions for sciatica including heat, massage, bed rest, dietary alterations, and soothing music. Later physicians became progressively more aggressive in their therapies. In the seventh century, Paul of Aegina recommended burning the hip joint at three or four places if conservative management failed. In the early tenth century, the famous Persian physician, Rhazes, claimed to successfully treat 1000 cases of sciatica in Baghdad with prolonged bleeding of the lower extremity. Even with the improved understanding of sciatica mechanisms in the nineteenth and early twentieth century, aggressive treatments continued to be popular including counter irritants (brine, wet cupping, and blistering) and a long list of physical agents (hydrotherapy, electrotherapy, ionic therapy, and even x-rays and radium as they became available). Only the rare patient survived treatment of sciatica unscathed.

Evidence Based Treatments

The current trend in medical practice is to develop so-called evidence-based guidelines for deciding on treatments. Ideally, this means following the results of carefully designed controlled treatment trials in large numbers of patients. However, since sciatica has so many causes and since there have been so few well designed treatment trials, it has been difficult to develop universally accepted management strategies. In such a situation, a doctor's training and experience determine the type of treatment that will be recommended. Regardless of the lack of high quality evidence, beginning in 1987, physicians around the world began developing guidelines for the initial management of sciatica based on evidence available at the time. The

© Springer International Publishing AG, part of Springer Nature 2019
R. W. Baloh, *Sciatica and Chronic Pain*,
https://doi.org/10.1007/978-3-319-93904-9_4

goal was to improve health care quality and reduce ineffective treatments. There was a general consensus that the prevailing approach at the time consisting of bed rest and regular use of pain medications did not work and in fact it prolonged recovery.

The first step with current evidence based guidelines for treating sciatica is to identify "red flags", findings that would require immediate referral to a specialist and imaging of the spine (see Table 3.1). After eliminating red flags, which are found in only a small percentage of people with sciatica, the rest are followed with conservative management for up to 6 weeks. Disabling symptoms resolve spontaneously within 6 weeks in the majority of people with sciatica. The guidelines recommend that people with new onset sciatica continue with routine activities as much as possible and use pain medications only as needed. The intent of the guidelines is to change the care focus to improve activity tolerance and avoid "unnecessary" diagnostic tests and treatment interventions. After reviewing all of the medical studies available committees on guidelines around the world concluded that intensive diagnostic and management approaches in people with new onset sciatica such as CT, MRI, injections, and surgery may actually prolong disability compared to benign management approaches.

There are multiple options for conservative management of people with new onset sciatica (Table 4.1) but little scientific evidence for choosing one option over another. Guidelines for the initial management of sciatica vary around the world but there is a general consensus that patients should be encouraged to maintain activity and pain should be controlled as much as possible. Prolonged bed rest should be avoided. Each management option can help with recovery but each has potential complications and the old adage "do no harm" must always be considered when deciding on a treatment.

Table 4.1 Comparison of treatments for new onset sciatica

Treatment	Advantages	Disadvantages
Pain medications	Relatively effective, cheap, widely available	Regular use may increase pain sensitivity, possible addiction
Muscle relaxants	Relieves pain of muscle spasm, sedation	Does not relieve nerve pain, sedation may inhibit mobility
Liniments	May help burning pain, cheap, widely available	Not helpful for severe or shooting pain
Physical therapy	Help maintain mobility, relax and strengthen muscles	May initially aggravate pain
Chiropractic	Help maintain mobility, relax muscles	Sudden manipulations can aggravate nerve damage
Acupuncture	Activates body own pain control system	Variably effective

Pain Medications

Anti-inflammatory Drugs

Acetylsalicylic acid (aspirin) is the most widely used anti-inflammatory drug used for pain relief in the world. It was derived from salicylic acid, a component of an herbal extract from the bark of a number of trees including willow, poplar and cinchona trees. The Sumerians described remedies for treating pain using the bark of the willow tree on clay tablets more than 4000 years ago. Ancient Mesopotamian and Chinese cultures also used willow bark for treating pain. Willow bark powder later became a popular treatment for rheumatism and lumbago. It wasn't until the nineteenth century, however, before investigators identified salicytic acid as the active ingredient for relieving pain and inflammation in willow bark (named for salicin, the Latin word for willow). This work was driven by Napoleon Bonaparte's blockade of the European continent that interfered with the importation of willow and cinchona tree bark from South America.

Aspirin, acetaminophen, and non-steroidal anti-inflammatory drugs (NSAIDS) such as ibuprofen and naproxen all work at least in part by blocking the enzyme COX-2 which in turn blocks the production and release of prostaglandin, a major component of "inflammatory soup" present at the site of acute tissue injury. As noted in Chap. 2, inflammatory soup refers to a mixture of pain generating molecules released in the damaged tissue. The main problem with regular use of aspirin is irritation of the gastrointestinal tract and bleeding. Therefore, most physicians around the world recommend acetaminophen or NSAIDS as the first choice for treating new onset sciatica since these drugs are relatively safe and also readily available (Table 4.2). NSAIDS can also cause GI irritation and bleeding but the risk

Table 4.2 Pain medications commonly used for acute sciatica

Class	Drug	Dosage[a] (as needed)	Major side effects
Cox inhibitors	Acetaminophen (Tylenol)	650–1000 mg every 6 h	Liver damage
	Ibuprofen (Motrin, Advil)	400–800 mg every 6 h	Gastritis, bleeding
	Naproxen (Alieve)	500–1000 mg every 6 h	Gastritis, bleeding
Muscle relaxants	Diazepam (Valium)	5–10 mg every 6 h	Sedation
	Cyclobenzaprine (Flexeril)	5–10 mg every 8 h	Sedation
Opioids	Tramadol (ConZip, Ultram, Ultracet[b])	25–100 mg every 6 h	Drowsiness, nausea, constipation
	Hydrocodone (Vicodin[b])	5–10 mg every 6 h	Nausea, constipation, addiction
	Morphine (MS Contin, Astramorph)	15–30 mg every 4 h	Nausea, constipation, addiction

[a]Always start with lowest dose and use lowest effective dose
[b]Combined with acetominophen

is lower than with aspirin. Chronic use of high dose acetaminophen can lead to severe liver damage.

Corticosteroids ("steroids") are natural substances secreted by the adrenal gland that regulate a wide range of metabolic functions including all aspects of inflammation. Natural and synthetic corticosteroids inhibit all inflammatory mediators including prostaglandin. A course of oral corticosteroids is commonly used to treat new onset sciatica but studies have not found this treatment very helpful and prolonged use can lead to major systemic side effects including GI bleed and psychosis. Injecting steroids into the damaged area is more effective but not recommended in the initial management. This treatment will be discussed later in Chap. 6.

Opioids

Like willow bark, the Sumerians were the first people known to cultivate the opium poppy, which they called the joy plant. Through the middle ages opium was primarily used for recreational purposes. In the sixteenth century the Swiss German philosopher, alchemist and physician, Philippus von Hohenheim introduced the European medical community to opium in the form of laudanum, a mixture of alcohol and opium. Von Hohenheim, better known as Paracelsus, Latin for "equal to Celsus" (a well-known Roman physician), lectured in German rather than Latin so that common people could understand his ideas. In the seventeenth century, Thomas Sydenham, known as the English Hippocrates for his broad medical acumen, introduced a new laudanum preparation that he used not only to alleviate back pain and sciatica but also to treat a wide range of illnesses including a range of nervous disorders. His laudanum consisted of opium dissolved in sherry wine with added saffron, cinnamon and clove. As the popularity of laudanum rapidly spread addiction to laudanum became a major health issue in English society. Two of the many famous laudanum addicts were the fictional detective, Sherlock Holmes and the Victorian author, Thomas De Quincey, whose book *Confessions of an English Opium-Eater* is still considered one of the best books ever written on drug addiction.

It wasn't until the beginning of the nineteenth century that the major active ingredient in opium was discovered. A German pharmacist, Friedrich Sertürner, dissolved opium in acid and then neutralized it with ammonia to produce morphine, named after Morpheus, the Greek god of dreams. Morphine is ten times as potent as opium and it rapidly became the "miracle drug" of the nineteenth century. E. Merck and Company of Germany were the first to commercially manufacture morphine in 1827 and a worldwide addiction epidemic soon followed. Morphine was widely used to treat pain during the American civil war and many soldiers became addicted in the aftermath.

There is a general consensus that opioid drugs should be a second line pain medication for new onset sciatica and only used if the first line anti-inflammatory drugs are ineffective. Further they should only be used for a short time (a few days) to help mobilize a patient who otherwise can't get out of bed. Combination drugs such as Vicodin (hydrocodone and acetaminophen) and Ultram (tramadol and acetaminophen) are often used first since they are less addictive and have less side effects than the more potent opioids (Table 4.2). In the late twentieth century a wave of more potent synthetic opioids were manufactured: meperidine (Demerol), fentanyl (Duragesic), and oxycodone (OxyContin and Percoset). As with earlier opium derivatives, there was hope that these drugs might be less addictive but a spike in the number of addictions occurred after each drug was introduced just as had previously occurred with laudanum, morphine and heroin. Many became addicted to opioids after they were given a prescription for treating back pain and sciatica.

Cannabis (Marijuana, Indian Hemp)

As far back as 2735 B.C. Chinese Emperor, Shen Neng, used cannabis tea to treat painful conditions such as sciatica and gout. Ancient physicians in Asia and the Middle East used cannabis extracts to treat a wide range of painful disorders even for relieving pain associated with child birth. Recreational use of cannabis was also popular in these ancient civilizations and doctors warned that overuse could cause impotence and blindness. An Irish born physician educated at the University of Edinburg, William O'Shaughnessy, introduced Western medicine to the use of cannabis in a paper presented at the Medical and physical Society of Calcutta, India in 1839. O'Shaughnessy, an assistant surgeon in the East India Company, traveled throughout India and the Middle East and collected information on the medical uses of cannabis from local physicians. When he returned to England his findings caused a sensation as physicians in Europe and America tried the new "wonder drug" for treating a wide variety of difficult to treat painful disorders. Chemists struggled to identify the active ingredients from extracts of the plant and this was not achieved until well into the twentieth century.

Despite the claims of its ardent supporters, smoked cannabis is not very effective for treating the pain of new onset sciatica. Furthermore, adverse effects including bronchial irritation and intoxication are common even when using vaporizers. Similarly although the major active ingredient in cannabis, THC, and synthetic THC analogues have been useful for treating chronic nausea they have not been very effective for treating pain. Variable absorption and associated intoxication and a profound state of unease have limited their use. Drugs combining THC with other minor components of cannabis show promise for treating chronic pain (see Chap. 9).

Muscle Relaxants

Muscle spasm often accompanies acute sciatica so techniques used to relax muscles can be beneficial particularly in combination with pain medications. The use of heat and massage to treat muscle spasm with sciatica can be traced to ancient times.

Hippocrates and his followers recommended heat and massage to treat sciatica. Heat supplied by a heating pad over the affected muscle or massage of the muscle can help relieve the spasm. If one can feel the spasm placing a tennis ball on the floor and rolling back and forth on the ball over the muscle (like using a rolling pin) may relieve the spasm. It is important to avoid excessive heat or deep massage since it could injure the tissue and make the problem worse. Muscle relaxant medications such as diazepam (Valium), cyclobenzaprine (Flexeril) and methocarbamol (Robaxin) might provide some additional pain relief along with other pain medications but sedation limits their usefulness (Table 4.2).

Liniments

The term liniment is derived from the Latin word *linere* meaning to anoint. It refers to topical medications that are applied to the skin to relieve pain and muscle tightness. Liniments are rubbed in to create friction over the painful area. They have been used for treating back pain and sciatica since antiquity and were typically composed of an evaporating solvent such as alcohol or acetone, an analgesic such as camphor or capsaicin and a counterirritant such as turpentine. The Renaissance physician Paracelsus formulated the most widely used liniment, opodeldoc. The name, opodeldoc, was derived from the variety of aromatic plants he used in his recipe. Opodeldoc was made up of soap, alcohol, camphor and several herbal essences including wormwood. It became the prototype for all future liniments. Subsequently the humorous name Old Opodeldoc became synonymous with an old bumbling doctor.

The United States has a rich tradition in the use of liniments for treating rheumatism and lumbago. Opodeldoc was widely used in New England at the time of Edgar Allen Poe and Poe used the name Opodeldoc for a character in his short story "The literary life of Thingum Bob, Esq." A common liniment used in the western United States was snake oil which originally came from China where it was a common remedy for lumbago (Fig. 4.1). Presumably, it was brought to North America by Chinese laborers working on the Transcontinental Railroad. When rubbed on the skin of the buttock and thigh, snake oil brought relief to patients with lumbago or so it was claimed. The established medical community of the time ridiculed the claim and the term snake oil became a generic term for questionable medicine marketed as a miraculous cure for any medical condition. The snake oil salesman was part of Western lore depicted in the movies as a "doctor" with questionable credentials selling medicines, often snake oil, with an accomplice in the crowd providing a testimonial to the miraculous benefits of the medicine. A classic example was W. C. Fields in the 1940 movie, Poppy. The most popular brand of snake oil produced by Clark Stanley contained mineral oil, beef fat, turpentine, chili pepper, and camphor. How Mr. Stanley came to add chili pepper to his liniment is unclear since it wasn't present in earlier versions brought from China, but his snake oil may have worked because of capsaicin present in chili peppers.

Fig. 4.1 Label from
Stanley's snake oil
liniment claiming to cure
rheumatism and sciatica

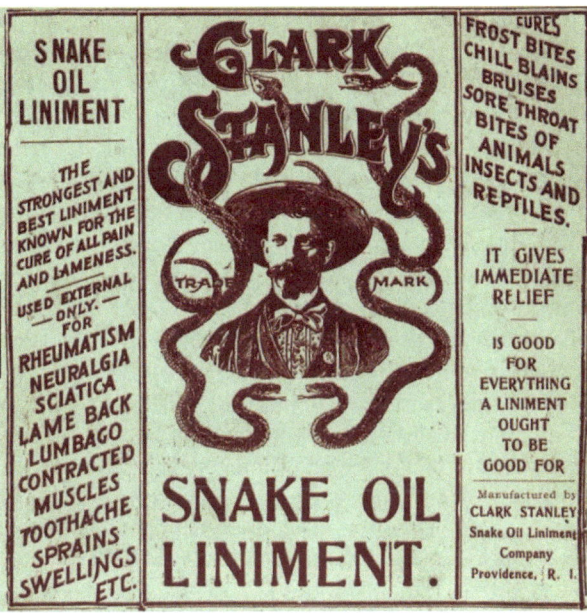

The fact that capsaicin is used for pain relief in a variety of liniments and ointments may seem like a paradox since capsaicin activates tiny pain receptors in nerve endings in the skin (see Chap. 2). Indeed when capsaicin is placed on the skin it initially causes burning pain but with time the burning disappears and the area becomes less sensitive to pain as the receptors in pain fiber terminals become desensitized. By applying a local anesthetic to the area prior to topical application of capsaicin the initial burning pain can be prevented. A variety of capsaicin patches are available (e.g. Qutenza, 8% capsaicin) in addition to many liniments containing capsaicin and the patches have been shown effective for treating nerve pain associated with shingles in controlled treatment trials. There are only anecdotal reports of beneficial effects for treating sciatica.

Physical Therapy

Physical therapy can trace its origin back to early Greek and Roman physicians who preached the importance of exercise, range of joint motions, massage and hydrotherapy for treating bone and joint diseases. American physical therapy began with World War I and the polio epidemic that followed. During the war a large group of women were recruited to help restore physical function to injured soldiers and they continued to treat polio patients and patients with other musculoskeletal disorders in the 1920s. Manual and mechanical traction became a major part of the treatment of acute sciatica as the importance of lumbar disc disease was demonstrated in the

1930s. The idea was that herniated discs could slip back into place if the vertebra above and below the ruptured disc were pulled apart by traction. Orthopedic surgeons and neurologists worked with physical therapists to develop a number of mechanical devices to provide traction to the lumbar spine with the goal of relieving spinal nerve compression. Although traction has been used for treating sciatic for hundreds of years there is little evidence that it works. A Cochrane Back Review Group analysis of controlled treatment trials for both mechanical and manual traction (just stretching the back), either alone or in combination with other treatments found that traction had little or no impact on pain intensity, functional status, global improvement and return to work among people with sciatica due to herniated discs. The Cochrane group is an international non-profit organization that generates systematic reviews of healthcare interventions.

In a similar review of controlled treatment trials, a structured exercise program with a physical therapist was found to be slightly better than just advice to remain active for reducing leg pain in the short term but no difference at intermediate and long-term follow-up between exercise and advice. Overall the evidence suggests that structured exercise has a small but significant effect on early improvement from new onset sciatica. Whether the effect is due to the therapy or simply "the laying on of hands" is difficult to say but of the various management options for new onset sciatica it is one the most cost effective and generally well received by patients and when performed appropriately is safe.

Alternative Medicine Techniques

Spinal Manipulations and Adjustments

Spinal manipulations and adjustments for treating back pain and sciatica date back as far as recorded medical history. In ancient Babylon, healers kneaded or struck the back while repeating the incantation "it shall be good." This manipulation employed to drive evil spirits out of the body no doubt occasionally caused the spine to pop or snap which was interpreted as a sudden exit of the unwanted spirit. Later, the notion of "a bone out of place" and "popping bones back into place" became the theoretical foundation for spinal manipulation and adjustments for treating back pain and sciatica.

Over the centuries, spinal manipulations and adjustments were carried out by a range of practitioners but in particular the practitioners of "bone setting". Bone setters also have an ancient tradition based on the notion that symptoms result from a dislocation of a bone or joint. Popping a dislocated shoulder or hip joint back into place no doubt had a dramatic impact on the suffering patient and the viewing public. Since the pain caused by other joint and bone diseases was similar to the pain associated with dislocation it is not hard to see how bone setters treated real and imagined joint and bone dislocation the same way. Lay bone setters were prevalent in England and early America. Probably best known in England was Sally Mapp, the daughter of a bone setter whose techniques had been developed in her family over centuries. "Crazy Sal" as she was known, toured London from her home in Epson setting bones and curing diseases.

In America in 1874, Andrew Taylor Still took the art of bone setting to a new level in developing the practice of osteopathy. Still believed that all diseases were caused by misplaced or maladjusted joints that interfered with nerve and blood supply. Proper manipulation of the joints cured the disease. About 20 years later, Daniel David Palmer founded chiropractic based on the belief that diseases were caused by misaligned vertebrae ("subluxations") that interfered with the transmission of what he called "Universal Intelligence" a kind spiritual energy that connected the brain to the rest of the body. He likened the subluxation to a "pinched hose." Palmer, a grocer in Davenport, Iowa who initially ventured into magnetic healing performed the first chiropractic adjustment on a janitor in 1895. Both Still and Palmer believed that their discoveries were based on divine intervention. Palmer compared himself to Christ, Mohammed, Smith, and other founders of religions. Their treatments appealed to the mainstream largely religious, poorly educated Americans of the time.

In the twentieth century, as scientific medicine became the foundation of medical practice, traditional osteopathy was abandoned and the practice of osteopathy adopted the same scientific principles as other medical fields. Chiropractic, however, was less willing to accept scientific methods and many chiropractors still maintain a metaphysical view of medical practice. Some "reform" chiropractors have tried to move toward more mainstream medical views advocating a limited use of chiropractic for treatment of musculoskeletal conditions. However, many chiropractors have found it difficult to shed their historical baggage. They still treat patients with sciatica with manipulations even though there is no scientific evidence that "subluxations" of the spine can cause sciatica or that manual manipulation corrects the "subluxation" if such a thing exists. Furthermore there is a real danger that manipulations can aggravate the nerve injury causing sciatica.

Why then are chiropractors treating so many patients with sciatica? Interestingly, when patients with low back pain and sciatica are surveyed, many prefer the care they received from chiropractors over that received from medical doctors. Chiropractors usually spend more time with patients than physicians do. They provide simple explanations that appeal to many patients and they take advantage of the remarkable healing power of "the laying on of hands". Medicare and medical insurance companies see these surveys and the lower costs of chiropractic treatment versus traditional medical treatment and they are happy to pay chiropractors for their services.

Acupuncture

Acupuncture is another ancient medical treatment for back pain and sciatica. The practice of acupuncture in China dates back at least 3000 years. It is based on the belief that good health requires a balance between yin and yang that depends on a subtle energy called Qi (pronounced "chee") that circulates through the body along channels called meridians. The medical practitioner can palpate Qi as it flows through the meridians and diagnose medical disorders. Treatment of abnormalities in the flow of Qi can be achieved with diet, exercise, massage, and insertion of thin metal needles at control points along the meridians. Terms such as dampness, wind, fire, dryness, cold and earth describe a person's state of health. If Chinese medicine resembles anything in the West, it would be the prescientific but rational Greek humoral medical system, which also perceived health states in such images of weather as phlegmatic (cold-moist) and choleric (hot-dry).

The origin of acupuncture is unclear but it may have been related to early bamboo or bone needles used for blood letting or providing an exit for evil spirits. Similarly there is little information on how the acupuncture points were originally identified but the anatomical locations of these points can be traced back to the stone age. Well preserved mummies from 5000 years ago were found to have non-ornamental tattoos in locations that correspond to traditional Chinese and modern acupuncture points. The 5200-year-old iceman, a.k.a. Otzi, found in the Tyrolean alps in 1991 had tattoo crosses on his back and foot that correspond with known acupuncture points commonly used to treat back pain and sciatica. Radiological studies of the Iceman showed severe arthritic changes in the low back, hips and knees. The tattoos could have provided a guide for self treatment of back pain. If so a form of acupuncture was being practiced in central Europe more than 5000 years ago.

French missionaries introduced Oriental medicine to Europe in the eighteenth century. Doctors picked up the technique of acupuncture and used it along with homeopathy that was popular at the time. An article published in the New York Times in 1972 by the journalist, James Reston stimulated American interest in acupuncture. He described how acupuncture relieved his pain during an emergency appendectomy that he underwent while accompanying President Nixon to China. Reston described how he watched patients undergoing surgery with only acupuncture for anesthesia. The patients talked throughout the procedure and when the surgery was over, they got up and walked back to their room.

Both acupuncture and chiropractic manipulations for treatment of sciatica have been evaluated in multiple placebo controlled treatment trials over the past several decades. A placebo is a drug or a procedure that has no known therapeutic benefit used as a control in a study to determine the effectiveness of a specific treatment. Placebos are also sometimes used by physicians to reinforce a patient's desire to get well. Some studies have found a significant benefit for acupuncture and chiropractic manipulations compared to placebo but critical reviews conclude that there is insufficient evidence to determine whether they are superior to placebo due to the study design. A major problem is how do you blind the therapist to avoid performance bias. Obviously the therapist knows which is the sham and which is the true procedure. Furthermore, how can a knowledgeable therapist perform a sham procedure that is identical in appearance and sensation to the real thing? Complicating matters further, all controlled trials of drugs and procedures for treating pain have a high placebo response rate meaning a high percentage of patients report improvement in pain from placebo treatment. Placebos probably relieve pain at least in part by activating the endogenous opioid system that blocks pain transmission in the spinal cord and brain (see Chap. 7). They work best when you "believe" they will work.

Overview of the Management of New Onset Sciatica

In summary, the key decision for managing new onset sciatica is whether or not red flags are present (Fig. 4.2). When red flags are identified, patients should be referred to a physician who specializes in spine disease and should undergo imaging of the back (usually MRI). If there are no red flags then conservative management is recommended for 6 weeks. If symptoms progress or red flags develop during the 6 weeks then referral to a specialist and imaging are required. Although multiple conservative management options are available (Table 4.1), current evidence supports the initial use of acetaminophen or ibuprofen every 6 h as needed and advice to remain active as much as possible. A structured exercise program with a physical therapist is probably better than just advice to remain active at least in the short term.

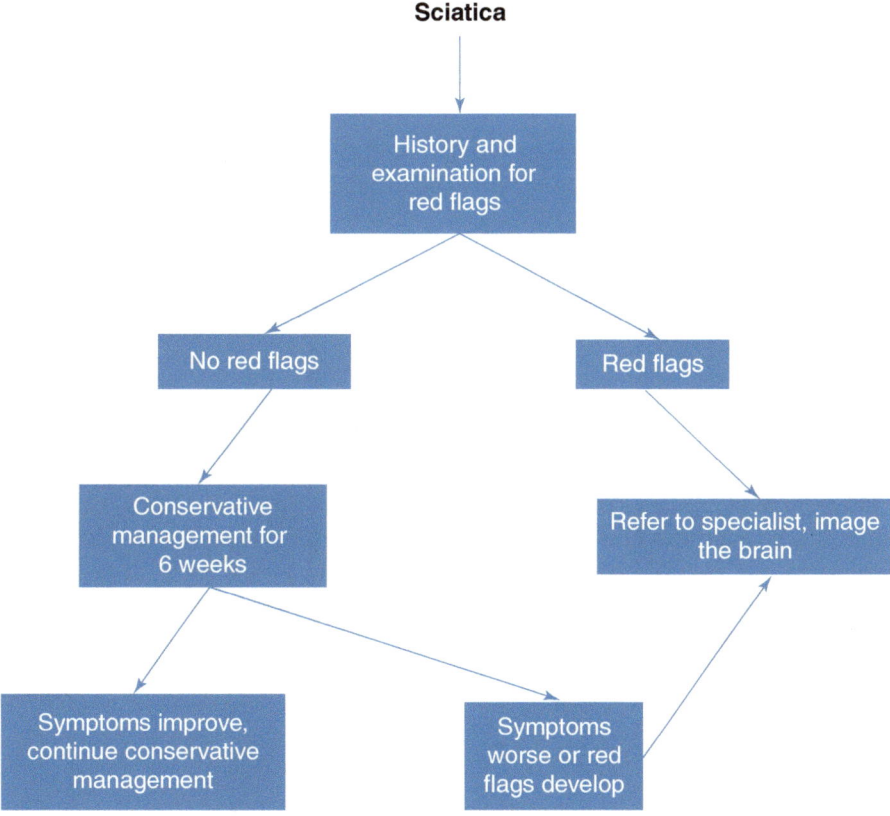

Fig. 4.2 Flow chart for management of new onset sciatica

Illustrative Cases Continued

Case 1

Since Alfredo continued to be bothered by pain despite regular use of ibuprofen his primary care physician gave him a prescription for Vicodin (hydrocodone and acetaminophen) one or two tablets every 6 h as needed. When he returned to see her 2 weeks later he reported that he was improving and able to carry on some normal activities including driving by taking two Vicodin every 6 h but he didn't feel as though he could return to work. He still had a positive straight leg raising sign on the right and walked slowly with a slightly bent forward posture. Alfredo had seen a chiropractor for back pain in the past with some success so he asked his primary care physician if he could see the chiropractor for treatment of his sciatica. He belonged to an HMO so he needed a referral from his primary care physician. She immediately requested and obtained approval for five visits with a chiropractor from the insurance company and she authorized three refills on his Vicodin prescription.

Comment

It was reasonable to give Alfredo Vicodin on his initial visit because his pain was restricting his routine activities but there should have been a plan to taper the Vicodin and replace it with a non-opioid drug and a discussion of the dangers of addiction with regular use of Vicodin. Although most insurance companies will pay for chiropractic treatment of sciatica there is no scientific evidence that it is effective and it can aggravate the condition.

Case 2

The team sport physician initially gave Lamar ibuprofen for pain relief and instructed him to avoid all activities that exacerbated the pain including any of his training exercises. The ibuprofen relieved the baseline continuous pain but he still had severe pain with any kind of activity. He was able to return to classes but he found that prolonged sitting also aggravated the pain. He was set up to see the team orthopedic surgeon, fitted with a back brace with the goal of stabilizing the spine and he was started on a physical therapy program consisting of core strengthening and stretching exercises.

Comment

Although bracing the back would seem a logical treatment for spondylosisthesis, as in the case of spinal traction for disc disease, controlled studies have not found a clear benefit for back exercises with bracing over back exercises without bracing. Probably, it simply is not possible to stabilize the vertebral column with an external brace. Furthermore, prolonged bracing can result in muscle atrophy.

Case 3

For the first few weeks, ibuprofen 400 mg every 6–8 h helped control my pain and I was able to carry on all my normal activities except tennis. My primary care physician arranged a course of physical therapy with two sessions a week during which the therapist worked on improving the range of motion and strengthening of the muscles in my low back. He also gave me a series of flexion exercises used for treating foramen and spinal stenosis that I performed twice a day at home. These consisted of sitting on a chair and bending forward placing open hands flat on the floor for ten repetitions and standing and bending forward to touch my toes for ten repetitions. But then I began having stomach problems with stomach pain and nausea. I tried acetaminophen but it wasn't very effective. After discussing the matter with my primary care physician we decided to try celecoxib (Celebrex), a newer selective COX-2 inhibitor that does not irritate the stomach. I received reasonable pain relief from the celecoxib and the terrible stomach ache and nausea went away. Another advantage of the celecoxib was that it lasted longer so I only needed to take it every 12 h.

Comment

I was following the recommended guidelines for initial management of sciatica by maintaining regular activities and using ibuprofen as needed for pain relief. The physical therapy program seemed a reasonable addition with little risk. The rationale for the flexion exercises is that repetitive flexion of the spine may "open up" the narrowed foramen relieving pressure on the spinal nerve. The main side effect of regular use of ibuprofen is irritation of the lining of the stomach thought to be due to blockage of COX-1, an enzyme that that protects the lining of the stomach and intestines. The newer selective COX-2 inhibitor celecoxib does not irritate the stomach but may have other long-term side effects (see Chap. 8).

Suggested Additional Reading

Booth M. Opium: a history. London: Simon & Schuster, Ltd.; 1996.
Jeffreys D. Aspirin: the remarkable story of a wonder drug. New York: Bloomsbury; 2005.
Kaptchuk TJ. The web that has no weaver: understanding Chinese medicine. 2nd ed. Lincolnwood: McGraw-Hill; 2000.

Chapter 5
Imaging the Back and Sciatic Nerve

We have come a long way in developing imaging procedures to diagnose sciatica in the past 40 years. When I began practicing neurology in the mid 1970s physicians and patients alike dreaded the procedures used to image the spine. The tests were difficult to interpret, were often very painful and could lead to permanent damage to the spinal cord and nerves. All this changed with the development of computed tomography (CT) in the late 1970s and magnetic resonance imaging (MRI) in the 1980s.

The German physicist Wilhelm Conrad Roentgen discovered X-rays in 1895 but it wasn't until after the turn of the twentieth century that technology advanced enough to generate good quality pictures of the back. X-rays are ultra-short electromagnetic waves that penetrate the body and are absorbed at different rates by tissues of different density. Early X-rays of the back took at least 15–30 min and it was difficult to focus the x-ray beam. X-rays were mainly useful for identifying bone fractures, bony displacements, or calcified tumors. There was not enough contrast density between the spinal cord, the spinal nerves and the spinal fluid to visualize these structures with X-rays. The next big advance in imaging the back was to combine x-rays with a contrast agent in the spinal fluid (such as air or a radiopaque dye) to outline the spinal cord and the sheaths of the spinal nerves as they exited the spine.

In the early 1920s a French physician, Jean Sicard first used iodized poppy seed oil, known as Lipiodol, as a contrast agent with X-rays to study the soft tissue structures of the back. At the time Lipiodol was a popular drug for treating a variety of conditions including syphilis, leprosy and nerve injuries. Sicard had been using it to treat sciatica by injecting it around the nerve in the pelvis or into the space around the lumbar dural sac (the epidural space). One of his students accidently penetrated the dura and injected it into the spinal fluid. Secard X-rayed the patient's lumbar spine and noted that the Lipiodol descended to the bottom of the dural sac nicely outlining the bottom of the spinal cord and the sheaths of the spinal nerves (see Fig. 3.1a). Because of its high iodine content (40%) Lipiodol provided a good contrast between the spinal fluid and the spinal cord and nerves on X-rays. There were

© Springer International Publishing AG, part of Springer Nature 2019
R. W. Baloh, *Sciatica and Chronic Pain*,
https://doi.org/10.1007/978-3-319-93904-9_5

problems however, in that most patients had pain for a few days after the procedure and some went on to develop inflammation of the arachnoid membrane surrounding the spinal cord and spinal nerves. Lipiodol was the only contrast agent available at the time Mixter and Barr published their famous 1934 article on lumbar disc surgery (see Chap. 3) and as the number of surgeries for disc disease increased exponentially the reports of side effects from Lipiodol also increased exponentially. Later, techniques were developed to suck the Lipiodol out of the spinal canal after the procedure but these techniques also had problems including extreme pain and occasional damage to the nerves and spinal cord. It wasn't until the 1970s that water soluble contrast agents were developed with the most popular being metrizamide that was absorbed into the blood stream so there was no need to remove it at the end of the procedure.

Early forms of X-ray tomography in which the X-ray source and film were rotated about a defined plane within the patient were developed in the early 1900s to focus on subtle bony changes such as a tiny fracture or bony erosion. Only the plane of interest was in focus with surrounding structures blurred. These were crude devises that did not provide the resolution necessary to visualize soft tissue structures within the bony spinal column. In 1961, William Oldendorf, a neurologist at the UCLA affiliated Wadworth VA Hospital in Los Angeles, published a brief report outlining a simple method to reconstruct the internal points of a three-dimensional object and portray them in a cross-sectional plane. Oldendorf was a practicing neurologist who had performed many contrast X-ray procedures and he was fed up with these painful crude tests that provided only limited information. He made his device in his basement using junk parts including his son's electric train and an old turntable. He used a radioactive source for radiation rather than X-rays but otherwise demonstrated the general principle and the hardware of modern CT scanners. Oldendorf patented his device but was unable to convince any of the X-ray machine manufacturers that he contacted to produce it. They didn't think it would be profitable.

A limitation of Oldendorf's publication was the lack of mathematical details regarding how the calculations would be made. He was a physician without a mathematical background and of course computers were in their infancy. A few years later a South African-born naturalized American, Alan Cormack published two papers describing the mathematical equations needed to reconstruct a cross-sectional plane from a three-dimensional object. It would be several years before Godfrey Hounsfield, an English engineer working at the Research Laboratory of Electrical and Music Industries (EMI), suggested that Cormack's mathematical technique could be used to reconstruct the internal structure of the body from X-ray transmission measurements. In his initial device made at EMI he used a radioactive source for radiation like Oldendorf but he later substituted an X-ray tube for the source. Early CT scans of a human brain took 9 h to complete but Hounsfield gradually improved the device working with radiologists and the first CT scanner was installed at the Atkinson Morley Hospital at Wimbledon in 1971. Hounsfield's CT scanner was large enough for the head only but the following year Robert Ledley, an American dentist with an MA in physics, developed the first body scanner. Ledley, built his original scanner with the help of a local automobile dealership. Cormack and Hounsfield received the Nobel Prize for their work in 1979 but Oldendorf was overlooked.

Magnetic resonance spectroscopy was used as far back as the 1940s to determine the chemical composition and structure of molecules. An American chemist, Paul Christian Lauterbur, was professor at the State University of New York at Stony Brook from 1963 to 1985 during which he built the first MRI machine. He would go on to share the Nobel prize in 2003 with the English physicist, Peter Mansfield for their work on MRI. As a teenager Lauterbur built a chemistry laboratory in the basement of his house. He later recalled that while he was a graduate student at the University of Pittsburgh the idea for the MRI came to him one day at a suburban Big Boy restaurant and he quickly scribbled it on a napkin. In his doctoral thesis he showed how introducing gradients in a magnetic field allowed one to identify the origin of radio waves emitted from nuclei of the object being studied. Some of the first images taken by Lauterbur's MRI machine, which is currently located in the Chemistry building at Stony Brook, included a small clam his daughter found on the beach and containers with ordinary water (H_2O) and heavy water (D_2O). This was the first imaging technique that could distinguish between these two varieties of water, an important point since most of the human body is made of water. Mansfield performed the mathematics showing how the radio signals from MRI could be made into a useful image. He also went on to show how one could use MRI to create much faster images a finding that made functional magnetic resonance images (fMRIs) possible. This is a type of MRI that visualizes blood flow and glucose uptake from the blood in real time. Unlike Lauterbur, Mansfield got a late start in schooling and was told at an early age that science was not for him. After returning from military service, however, he gained entrance to Queen Mary College in London where he studied physics and was part of a project to study the Earth's magnetic field which initiated his interest in MRI.

Strategy for Imaging the Back in Patients with Sciatica

As noted in Chap. 4, there is general agreement that the back should be imaged in people with sciatica who exhibit "red flags" or if their pain persists or progresses beyond 6 weeks of conservative management. There are multiple imaging options to identify the cause of sciatica and each has advantages and disadvantages (Table 5.1) but most would agree that the procedure of choice in most cases is an MRI of the lumbar spine (Fig. 5.1). MRI provides the best contrast between bone and soft tissues and provides the best visualization of the spinal cord and spinal nerves. Routine X-rays are relatively cheap (about $50 compared to $300–1000 for an MRI of the low back), but compared to MRI they are not very sensitive. As noted earlier they can identify vertebral bone fractures and developmental or degenerative changes in the bony spine but do not visualize the spinal nerves or sciatic nerve. Modern computerized X-ray scans (C-T scans) give much better images of the bone

Table 5.1 Comparison of procedures for imaging the back

Imaging procedure	Advantages	Disadvantages
X-ray of lumbar spine	Can identify bone fractures, displacement and erosion; fast, cheap and widely available	Cannot visualize discs, tumors, nerve compression or nerve entrapment
CT of lumbar spine	Can visualize bony abnormalities, facet joints and discs; fast, relatively cheap and widely available	Cannot visualize nerve compression; radiation exposure
CT of pelvis	Can visualize tumors, abscesses and blood in the pelvis	Cannot visualize nerve compression or entrapment; radiation exposure
MRI of lumbar spine	Can visualize degenerative disc disease and evidence of nerve compression; no radiation exposure	Ferromagnetic problems, claustrophobia
MRI Neurography of the pelvis	Can visualize nerve compression or entrapment in the pelvis, no radiation exposure	Ferromagnetic problems, claustrophobia, can take up to 45 min

Fig. 5.1 Magnetic resonance image (MRI) of the lumbosacral spine in a normal 60 years old subject (lateral view). Compare with the anatomy shown in Fig. 3.1a. In this T_2 sequence, spinal fluid (white) outlines the bottom of the spinal cord at the T12-L1 level and the spinal nerves in the cauda equina

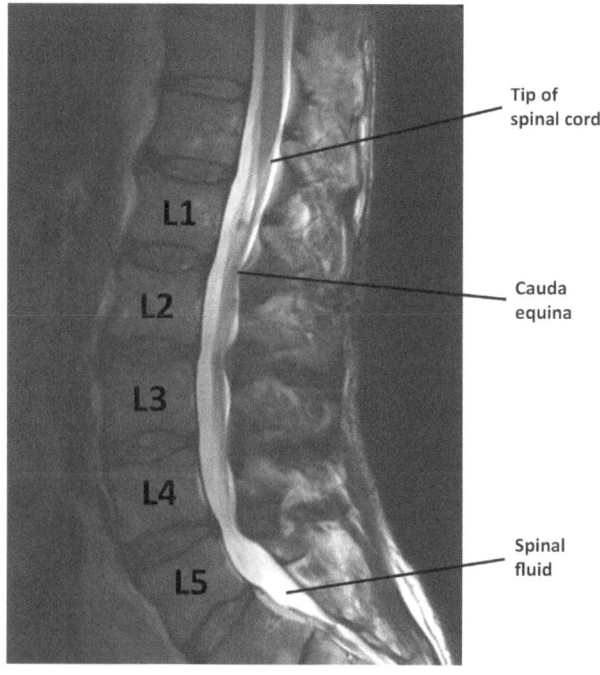

and herniated discs than routine X-rays but still can not compare with MRI for imaging the spinal cord and spinal nerves. CT or MRI of the spine after intravenous contrast dye injection can identify vascular anomalies and small vascular tumors such as schwannomas that might be missed without the contrast agent (see Fig. 5.2).

If images of the lumbar spine do not identify the cause of sciatica then the focus should be on the pelvis and sciatic nerve. The pelvis is the area between the hips that contains the reproductive organs, several important muscles including the piriformis muscle, the spinal nerves that form the sciatic nerve and the sciatic nerve itself. C-T and MRI of the pelvis are about equally effective for identifying pelvic tumors, abscesses and hemorrhage but MRI provides the best visualization of the soft tissue structures. MRI neurography is a new technology that is rapidly becoming the procedure of choice for identifying compression, inflammation or entrapment of the spinal nerves and sciatic nerve within the pelvis (see Fig. 5.3).

Fig. 5.2 MRI of the lumbosacral spine showing three schwannomas involving the cauda equine (lateral view). The largest tumor at the L2 level is about 1.2 cm in diameter. In this T_1 sequence the contrast enhanced tumors are easily seen. The spinal fluid is black with this sequence

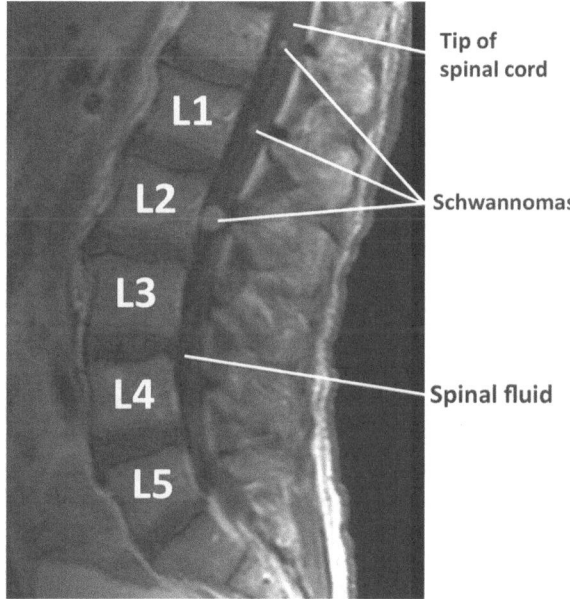

Fig. 5.3 MRI of the pelvis showing the sciatic nerves running beneath the prirformis muscles (P) without evidence of compression (horizontal view). The piriformis muscle on the right was smaller than the muscle on the left

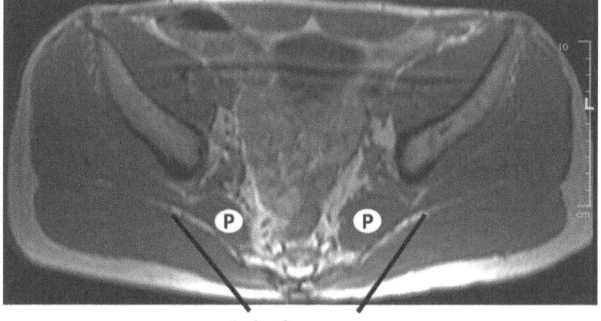

Overview of Current Techniques for Imaging the Back

Routine X-Rays of the Spine

The main advantages of standard X-rays of the spine are that they are quick, cheap and widely available. They are of little use, however, for routine screening of people with new onset sciatica since they will not identify the vast majority of causes. They can be useful for initial evaluation in young athletes with possible spine fracture and dislocation and X-ray machines are often available at sporting events. Since X-rays can be obtained with the subject standing it is easy to evaluate the effect of body position such as bending backwards on the vertebral bone dislocation. Most chiropractors routinely order spine X-rays to look for "subluxations" before treating their patients with sciatica. As noted in Chap. 4, however, subluxations can be seen in anyone and there is no scientific evidence that subluxations cause sciatica or any other symptoms. Paradoxically, Medicare requires chiropractors to document subluxations with X-rays of the spine to justify their manipulations.

Computed Tomography (CT) of the Spine and Pelvis

Like a routine X-ray, a CT scan of the spine is relatively quick, cheap and widely available compared to MRI but it is not very good for assessing the fine structure of soft tissues. It is ideal for evaluating bone fractures and displacements and it can reliably identify ruptured discs but not whether they are compressing nerves. It is ideal for visualizing degenerative changes in the facet joints. CT of the pelvis readily identifies tumors, abscesses and bleeding but doesn't show if the sciatic nerve is being compressed. A CT of the spine results in the radiation equivalent of about 640 chest X-rays so radiation exposure can become a problem with multiple repeat studies.

Magnetic Resonance Imaging (MRI) of the Spine and Sciatic Nerve

As noted previously MRI of the spine is the "gold standard" for imaging the back in people with sciatica and it is the only technique that allows a direct visualization of the spinal and sciatic nerves. Furthermore there is no radiation exposure. The large magnet used for MRI can cause problems if you have metal in your body such as a pacemaker, metal plates, screws or clips from prior surgery or an artificial heart valve. Most current MRIs are performed with the subject enclosed in a hollow tube so claustrophobia can also be a problem. However, open upright MRI scanners are becoming widely available and these newer scanners can image the back while the patient is siting, standing straight and bending forward or backward. Many of the common causes of sciatica are relieved or aggravated in certain body positions. MRI neurography has been particularly useful for identifying nerve entrapment in the pelvis such as with the piriformis syndrome (see Chap. 3). Enlargement of the muscle and swelling of the nerve can be identified and response to treatment can be documented.

Illustrative Cases Continued

Case 1

The chiropractor agreed that Alfredo had sciatica and arranged for X-rays of the lumbar spine in his office. He showed Alfredo the X-rays pointing out two slight misalignments of lumbar vertebrae (subluxations) and indicated that the misalignments were interfering with nervous control of his right leg. He recommended a series of manipulations to improve the misalignments and when Alfredo agreed, he immediately began the first treatment. The pain was slightly worse for a day or so after each treatment but his chiropractor reassured him that this was not unusual. When there was a sudden worsening of pain after his fourth treatment session, however, the chiropractor recommended that he should probably undergo an MRI of the lumbar spine. At this point Alfredo's primary care physician requested and obtained approval for an MRI of the lumbar spine and a referral to an orthopedic surgeon that specialized in back problems.

Alfredo's MRI of the lumbar spine took about 25 min. He was given ear plugs to dampen the loud sounds of the machine and told to hold perfectly still for several three minute sequences. Fortunately, he was not claustrophobic but that could have been a problem since he was completely enclosed in a long narrow tunnel. When he saw the orthopedic surgeon a few days later he was told that there was a large disc herniation pressing on a nerve going to his right leg and that the MRI showed that the nerve and surrounding tissue was swollen and inflamed.

Comment

It is difficult to know whether the chiropractic manipulations aggravated Alfredo's condition since sciatica associated with disc herniation can persist regardless of treatment but clearly the manipulations did not help his condition. Since his symptoms persisted despite conservative treatment it was time for imaging of his back and referral to a specialist. The MRI documented a disc herniation and evidence of continued nerve inflammation so other treatment options such as injections or surgery had to be considered.

Case 2

The university sports doctor initially ordered X-rays with front and side views of the lumbar spine while Lamar was standing straight, bending forwards and bending backwards. The study identified a fracture of the pars interarticularis, the key bone that stabilizes the back of the spine. In addition there was a slight slippage forward of the L5 vertebra on the S1 vertebra that appeared to increase when Lamar bent backwards and decrease when he bent forwards. The doctor made a diagnosis of mild spondylolisthesis due to the spinal fracture and advised Lamar to stop all exercise, use ibuprofen as needed for pain and to continue physical therapy with stretching the back. Four weeks later Lamar continued to have pain in the back and in both legs and he was concerned that he was getting weak because of lack of exercise. The sports physician decided to order an MRI of the lumbar spine and refer Lamar to a neurosurgical colleague. The MRI documented the fracture and the forward slippage of the L5 vertebra and in addition showed likely compression of the L5 and S1 spinal nerves on both sides.

Comment

Routine X-rays were useful in this case since they can identify bone fracture and vertebral body displacement and they can be performed with the patient standing and bending forward and backward. Furthermore, they are available at many sporting facilities. The MRI allowed visualization of the spinal nerve compression and a precise measurement of the amount of translation between the L5 and S1 vertebral bodies, in this case found to be about 40%. Under 50% is considered low-grade displacement while over 50% is high-grade displacement. Most people with low grade displacement do eventually recover without the need for surgery but the combination of the MRI findings of multiple spinal nerve compressions was worrisome.

Case 3

It was nearly 5 weeks since the onset of my pain and it was gradually getting worse but I continued to work and exercise lightly. But then a new symptom developed that changed everything. I began awakening in the middle of the night with severe pain in the buttock that forced me to get up and move around. Once the pain started I could not find any position that was comfortable and I had to get up to obtain relief. I tried increasing the dose of celecoxib to no avail and I began sleeping in a recliner for some relief but I still could not sleep through the night. When I told my primary care physician about this new symptom he immediately put in a request for an MRI of the lumbar spine and a referral to neurosurgery. The MRI was scheduled for the next day but I would have to wait a week for the consult.

After the MRI was complete, I walked over to the neuroradiology department to go over the images with our neuroradiologist. As I arrived, he had my MRI images on his computer screen. "I think we have the answer," he said as he pointed at a small area of narrowing (stenosis) of the bony foramen in the lower lumbar spine on the left side. The fifth lumbar spinal nerve was touching the bony protrusion but it wasn't clearly compressed or inflamed. The rest of the spine looked good except for degenerative changes not unexpected in someone of my age. "Your pain is on the left side, right?" he asked. My heart sank. My pain was on the right side.

Comment

We had come upon a common problem when using MRI to identify the cause of sciatica. It can be too sensitive. A wide range of changes in bone, intervertebral discs and ligaments can be identified in normal people with MRI including bulging discs, degenerative arthritic changes and even occasionally a ruptured disc. In order to be sure that the osteoarthritis or disc protrusion is the cause of sciatica, there should be evidence of nerve compression or inflammation on MRI and it should be in the correct location to explain the pain symptoms. Not infrequently, patients undergo surgery to treat MRI findings that have nothing to do with their symptoms. No wonder there is controversy about treatment results for sciatica and why many recommend no treatment at all (other than pain medication).

Case 3 Continued

The neuroradiologist discussed my MRI findings with the neurosurgeon that I was scheduled to see and they agreed that I should go ahead and have MRI neurography of the pelvis to rule out compression or entrapment of a spinal nerve in the pelvis. In the meantime, the neuroradiologist informed me that he reviewed my low back MRI in more detail and thought there might be an "irregularity" at the L2 level within the dural sac and even though this didn't seem to explain my sciatica, he felt that we should repeat a lumbar spine sequence with contrast dye. The second MRI with contrast and neurography took much longer, over an hour, and I noticed that lying on the hard MRI table markedly aggravated my pain. But I didn't move because I wanted clear pictures. Again I walked over to neuroradiology and we looked at the images together. First the sciatic nerves in the pelvis looked normal without any evidence of compression (Fig. 5.3). The piriformis muscle on the right was even smaller than the muscle on the left. There was no evidence of piriformis spasm or sciatic nerve entrapment. To our surprise, the repeat study of the lumbar spine with contrast showed a round contrast-enhancing ball (about a half inch in diameter) attached to a spinal nerve at the L2 level on the right side (Fig. 5.2). We both felt that it had the typical features of a schwannoma, a benign tumor of the nerve sheath (see Chap. 3). Even more remarkable, there were two other tiny (pea sized) contrast-enhancing balls on other spinal nerves in the in the same region.

Comment

But how could a tumor at the L2 level cause sciatica with pain in the distribution of the L5 spinal nerve? Recall that the spinal cord ends at about the T12 level so that all of the lumbar and sacral spinal nerves exit at that level (see Fig. 3.1a). The tumor compressed the L5 spinal nerve at the L2 level as it made its way down the spinal canal to exit below L5. Pain in the L5 distribution would be the same regardless of where along its course it was damaged from just below the bottom of the spinal cord to where it joins together with the other spinal nerves to form the sciatic nerve in the pelvis (see Fig. 3.1b).

So now what do we do. I had a small grape size tumor and two pea size tumors on the spinal nerves in my low back. The MRI features were typical of schwannomas but one cannot be certain without examining the tissue. There are genetic disorders associated with multiple schwannomas throughout the body but I had no family history of schwannomas. Just to be sure, I had MRIs of the cervical and thoracic spine with contrast and no other schwannomas were found. This condition has been called segmental schwannomatosis, presumably a mutation occurs in a tumor suppressor gene late in development in just one segment of the developing nervous system. In other words, the mutation is not in the germ line. Since there are two copies of each gene, one from your mother and one from your father, a second random mutation must occur in the second copy of the tumor suppressor gene later in life as Schwann cells constantly divide and replace older cells. It is probably safe to say that many of us have a tiny schwannoma on a nerve somewhere in the body. Schwannomas are particularly common on the 8th cranial nerve, the hearing and balance nerve, where they typically present with slowly progressive hearing loss on one side. They represent about 10% of all brain tumors. About 3% of the general population has a tiny schwannoma on the eighth nerve on routine autopsies, most of which never became large enough to cause symptoms. Presumably in my case, the large tumor was responsible for my sciatic pain by compressing spinal nerves L4 and L5 and the other tiny tumors were asymptomatic.

Suggested Additional Reading

Dawson MJ. Paul Lauterbur and the invention of MRI. Boston: MIT Press; 2013.
Kraemer J, Koester O, Kraemer R, Schmid G. MRI of the lumbar spine: a teaching atlas. New York: Thieme; 2003.
Oldendorf WH. The quest for an image of the brain. New York: Raven Press; 1980.

Chapter 6
Anesthetics, Steroids and Surgery for Sciatica

There is little doubt that anesthetic and steroid injections can lead to dramatic pain relief in some patients with sciatica. Similarly, surgery can provide almost immediate relief of excruciating pain in some patients. As a rule, injections provide transient relief whereas surgery offers the possibility of a cure. The challenge is to determine the most effective treatment with the least likelihood of complications. Although we now have more than a century of experience with these treatments for sciatica there are still many unanswered questions.

Local Anesthetics and Steroids

South American natives chewed coca leaves for recreation and pain relief hundreds of years ago. Early European visitors brought back stories of the exceptional virtues of the coca plant and in 1859 the Italian, Paolo Mantegazza who lived in South America for many years, published his work on the medical uses of coca. In the same year the Austrian frigate *Novara* brought coca leaves back to Vienna and the alkaloid, cocaine was isolated from the leaves for the first time. Much of the early work was done through self-experimentation and many of the early experimenters became addicted to the drug. One of the early vigorous supporters of cocaine was Sigmund Freud who eventually became an addict. He was one of the first to emphasize the local anesthetic properties of cocaine when applied to the skin and mucous membranes particularly in the eye, mouth and larynx. In America, the New York surgeon William Stewart Halsted, began to experiment on himself and colleagues by injecting nerves with cocaine to produce rapid reversible local anesthesia. Halsted also became an addict. Cocaine was first injected in the epidural space to treat sciatica in 1901 but cocaine toxicity commonly occurred and pain relief was brief. Later safer derivatives of cocaine were developed for local anesthesia, first procaine in 1904, novocaine a year later and the most widely used local anesthetic agent, lidocaine in 1943. In addition to injecting peripheral nerves and the epidural

© Springer International Publishing AG, part of Springer Nature 2019   57
R. W. Baloh, *Sciatica and Chronic Pain*,
https://doi.org/10.1007/978-3-319-93904-9_6

space these anesthetic drugs were also injected into the spinal fluid to produce anesthesia below the level of the injection. Cocaine and its many derivatives work as
local anesthetics by blocking sodium ion channels in nerve fibers so that action
potentials moving along the nerve are blocked. Pain signals are not able to pass
through the block.

As noted in Chap. 4, corticosteroids are normally secreted by the adrenal gland
to control a wide range of metabolic activities including all aspects of inflammation.
The first synthetic coticosteroid, Compound E (cortisone), was discovered in 1936
followed by Compound F (hydrocortisone) in 1950; both were found useful for
treating a range of inflammatory conditions particularly arthritis. Steroids were first
injected in the epidural space just outside the dura to treat sciaitca in the mid 1950s
with the goal of obtaining high local concentration near the inflamed spinal nerve.
Other investigators injected the steroids inside the dural sac but complications were
frequent so epidural injections became the preferred technique.

Epidural Injections

Epidural steroids refers to the injection of steroids, usually mixed with a local anesthetic, into the space surrounding the lumbosacral dura to relieve pain due to inflammation of a spinal nerve (see Fig. 3.1a). The needle is typically placed under fluoroscopic
guidance to decrease the risk of complications. A variety of steroids and local anesthetics have been used but a popular combination is dexamethasone and bupivacaine.
Dexamethasone is a water-soluble steroid that does not aggregate and bupivacaine is a
relatively long acting local anesthetic. The drugs can be injected into the epidural space
or next to the affected spinal nerve. An immediate relief of pain helps confirm the location of the nerve injury and the diagnosis. Although local anesthetics alone provide
pain relief combining with steroids provides better long-term relief. A contrast agent
can be injected with the drugs to confirm that they have been directed to the target
nerve. Most responders receive short-term (weeks to months) pain relief. One study
found that about half of the patients with herniated discs randomly assigned to receive
epidural steroids had a good response. An even higher response rate is seen in patients
with foramen or spinal stenosis due to osteoarthritis. Some reports suggest a long lasting benefit in rare patients so that they are "saved" from surgery. Of course they may
just have had a spontaneous remission as the underlying process heals.

Epidural steroids are used to treat a variety of causes of sciatica: herniated discs,
osteoarthritic narrowing of a foramen, synovial cysts, fractures of the lumbar spine
and spinal stenosis. All of these are associated with inflammation of nerves and
nearby tissues. Absolute contraindications are hypersensitivity to the drugs including a contrast agent if used, local infection or malignancy, and a bleeding tendency.
They should be used with caution in patients with diabetes, heart failure, immune
suppression and pregnancy (because of risk to the fetus). Complications include
bleeding or infection at the site of injection, nerve injury from the needle, transient
numbness or weakness and fluid retention.

Injections for Nerve Entrapment

Steroids and local anesthetics can be injected near nerves in the pelvis that are entrapped by normal muscle or other tissue since there is typically inflammation of the nerve and surrounding tissue. The contraindications, risks, and complications are similar to those for epidural injections. This has been the procedure of choice for treating the pain with the piriformis muscle syndrome but controlled treatment trials are lacking. Although many physicians will insert the needle blindly based on the known location of the muscle in the pelvis the outcome is better and complications less if the needle insertion is guided by ultrasound or MRI. More recently there have been multiple reports of injecting botulinum toxin into the piriformis muscle to shrink the muscle and relieve the nerve entrapment. Botulinum toxin blocks nerve impulses to muscles causing them to atrophy. It is used for a wide range of neurological disorders including torticollis and strabismus. A few cases with the piriformis syndrome studied with MRI neurography before and after botulinum injections, documented lessening of the nerve inflammation and shrinkage of the piriformis muscle. The botulinum toxin effect is reversible after a few months but the syndrome may not recur.

Procedural Sedation

In the latter half of the twentieth century several relatively safe, rapidly acting intravenous anesthetic agents were developed and used for medical procedures. The two most commonly used agents are midazolam (Versed) and propofol (Diprivan). Patients are awake but sedated and typically have no recollection of the event after it is over (amnesia). Both of these drugs enhance inhibitory transmission in the brain and spinal cord but propofol also blocks sodium channels. Propofol is shorter acting (minutes) than midazolam (hours) so it is useful for brief procedures where longer sedation is undesirable. Both drugs are commonly combined with the opioid fentanyl for preoperative sedation. Some physicians use these drugs with epidural and piriformis muscle injections but others prefer to just use a local anesthetic injection in the skin prior to the procedure so that the patient can better report on the immediate effect of the injection.

General Anesthesia for Surgery

Today the thought of undergoing a major surgical procedure without anesthesia seems almost unimaginable. Yet such surgical procedures were routinely conducted without anesthesia well into the nineteenth century. Even when anesthetic agents became generally available there was surprising resistance to their use. Surgeons expressed concerns about operating on a "lifeless body" that could not react to pain. They were used to receiving feedback from the patient to guide them in their work. Some expressed concern that the patients were suffering even though they had no memory of the event. The French physiologist François Magendie was one of the most vocal critics of the use of general anesthetic agents. He felt that it was unethical to operate on a "dead drunk" patient (his description of a patient under anesthesia) since the patient was defenseless and potentially at the mercy of a "heavy-handed" surgeon. The conscious patient provided an important constraint on the surgeon's behavior. Magendie provided anecdotes where anesthesia triggered inappropriate erotic dreams in young women and changed normally reserved and bashful women into nymphomaniacs. Understandably these comments lead to a rauckous debate in the press and the academic community at the time.

Gaseous general anesthetics date back at least to the early sixteenth century when Paracelsus mixed sulfuric acid and alcohol and distilled the mixture to produce "sweet vitriol" or ether. Paracelsus noted that giving the substance to chickens put them to sleep and when given to patients it relieved pain without any apparent harm. It would be centuries later that the usefulness of ether anesthesia for surgery was appreciated, however. In the early 1800s ether "frolics" became very popular in the United States. People would do and say strange things under the influence of ether. In Georgia, a young physician, Crawford Long, who attended several ether frolics, noticed that one of the men at the frolic had two small tumors in his neck. Long asked the man if he would be willing to have his tumors removed while unconscious under ether. He agreed and on March 30th 1842, Long saturated a towel with ether, had the man breathe the ether and successfully removed the tumors with little pain. Long did several more surgeries with ether but waited until 1849 before publishing an article describing his experience. In the interval, William Morton, a Boston dentist began using ether in his dental practice and he developed an apparatus to administer the ether gas. He persuaded John Warren, a renowned surgeon at the Massachusetts General Hospital (MGH) in Boston, to use his ether machine in a demonstration operation to remove a tumor from a man's jaw at the main operating theatre. The skeptical audience marveled at the successful operation performed without pain. The MGH surgical operating theatre later became known as the "ether dome".

In 1831, an American physician and amateur chemist, Samuel Guthrie reacted chlorinated lime with ethanol to produce a compound that he thought was chlorinated ether or chloric ether. A few years later the French chemist Jean-Baptiste Dumas determined that the chemical structure of Guthrie's compound was trichloromethane which he named chloroform. Guthrie had suggested that the compound might be a good anesthetic agent but it wasn't until 1847 that a Scottish physician, James Young Simpson, used it in human subjects. Simpson first tried chloroform on two of his dinner guests for entertainment rather than medical purposes. A few days later a Scottish dentist, Francis Brodie Imlach was the first to use chloroform on a patient. The use of chloroform anesthesia rapidly expanded first in Europe and then in America because its onset of action was faster and it lasted longer than ether offering greater security of use. Its use got a great boost in popularity in the 1850s when it was used during the birth of Queen Elizabeth's last two children. However, with more widespread use it became apparent that there were a significant number of sudden deaths due to cardiac arrythmia in otherwise healthy people receiving chloroform. As other anesthetic agents became available in the twentieth century chloroform was largely abandoned because of its toxicity.

Most all of the modern gaseous anesthetic agents are chemical derivatives of ether and chloroform. Despite the use of gaseous anesthetics for more than a century and a half the mechanism of action of these drugs is still poorly understood. It is thought that the anesthetic gases are widely distributed in the brain where they interact with the lipid membrane of nerve cells and interfere with transmembrane proteins particularly ion channels that determine neuronal excitability. One theory is that they increase potassium influx through a class of potassium ion channels leading to hyperpolarization of neurons. These gaseous anesthetics clearly suppress pain perception and produce amnesia for the event.

Overall major risks of general anesthesia are small. Deaths occur in about 1 in 100,000 and serious side effects such as generalized allergy (anaphylaxis) or respiratory failure occur in about 1 in 10,000 patients undergoing general anesthesia. Less serious side effects such as nausea and vomiting, shivering, confusion and memory loss, bladder problems and sore throat and damage to the mouth and teeth from the endotracheal tube are more common. Most of these symptoms are transient, no more than a day or so, but some people will have persistent cognitive and memory impairment for days to months and rarely even years. The risk is much greater if patients have pre-existing cognitive and memory impairment and if they are over 70 years of age. Risks of side effects are also greater if there is a history of smoking, seizures, obstructive sleep apnea, hypertension and diabetes. Different anesthetic agents all seem to have similar rates of side effects but longer duration and deeper levels of anesthesia increase the risk of side effects particularly cognitive and memory impairment. Some older people will develop dramatic delirium with vivid hallucinations in the immediate postoperative period so it is important that family members are present and nursing staff is alerted.

Surgery for Sciatica

As noted earlier in this chapter, there is little doubt that surgery can dramatically cure some causes of sciatica. Surgery is the only effective treatment of tumors and abscesses compressing spinal nerves or the sciatic nerve. These disorders get worse despite conservative non-surgical management. Progressive compression of the cauda equina with resulting lower extremity weakness and bladder and bowel dysfunction requires immediate surgical exploration regardless of the cause. The benefit of surgical treatment for sciatica due to a herniated disc is less clear. There are many examples where a herniated disc is seen on MRI and the nerve compression is relieved by surgery and the patient immediately gets better. Like with penicillin, sometimes you only need one case to prove a treatment is effective. The result of surgery in other cases is not so clear, however, particularly in those with chronic sciatica due to longstanding disc disease. People with herniated discs usually get better with or without surgery and there is not a single controlled treatment trial comparing decompression surgery versus sham surgery for treating herniated discs (acute or chronic). Most would argue that it is unethical to ask patients to undergo sham surgery. But surgery can be a powerful placebo, the ultimate "laying on of the hands." The strong placebo effect of surgery is well documented in other surgical fields where surgery has been compared with sham surgery.

A laminectomy removes the bony lamina of the vertebra to get access to the spinal cord or the spinal nerves (see Fig. 3.3). Although there is some controversy regarding who was the first to perform a laminectomy, one of the first laminectomies was performed by the English surgeon, Victor Horsley. A 42 years old man presented to William Gowers, the famous English neurologist, with paralysis and loss of sensation in his legs. Gowers localized the problem to the mid thoracic spine based on his neurological examination and he convinced Horsley to operate. Horsley removed a benign tumor at the level of the third and fourth thoracic spinal nerves and the patient made a complete recovery.

Horsley, who had assisted in the first brain surgery in England the year before, was a remarkable character known for his operative speed and skills that minimized blood loss and anesthesia time, key to survival at that time. The American neurosurgical pioneer, Harvey Cushing, went to London with the notion of studying under Horsley, but changed his mind after a brief visit. Cushing, who was known for his meticulous behavior and surgical technique, obviously was not comfortable with Horsley's bravado. John Fulton, Cushing's biographer, described Cushing's impressions of Horsley as reported years later by one of Cushing's students. On arriving at Horsley's home, Cushing found a chaotic atmosphere with Horsley dictating letters to his secretary, eating breakfast and patting his dogs while talking with Cushing. Horsley offered to take Cushing with him to observe him perform surgery on the trigeminal nerve ganglion in a woman with chronic facial pain. This would be analogous to cutting a lumbosacral dorsal root ganglion for sciatica. They drove off in a cab after sterilizing Horsley's instruments and packing them in a towel. They arrived at an impressive West End mansion and Horsley ran upstairs, administered ether to the patient and was operating within 15 min of entering the house. Horsley made a large hole in the woman's skull, lifted up the temporal lobe and cut the trigeminal nerve at the sensory ganglion. He controlled the bleeding, closed the wound and they were out of the house in less than an hour from the time they entered.

Not only did Horsley develop novel neurosurgical techniques, he was a scientist and social reformer. As noted in Chap. 2, Horsley was the first to describe the tiny pain fibers in the sheaths of peripheral nerves that in part explains why compression of nerves is so painful. He was the first to record electrical charges in human peripheral nerves and in the spinal cord. This technique was a forerunner of modern electromyography (EMG) techniques used to monitor nerve electrical activity during spinal surgery. Horsley was a staunch supporter of women's rights, having fought for admission of women to medical school, nursing as a profession, and the suffragette movement. His passionate dislike for tobacco and alcohol alienated him to many of his peers, particularly those in the military. Horsley's career came to a tragic end when at age of 57 he volunteered for active duty during World War I and suffered a fatal heat stroke while stationed in Iraq.

The first laminectomy for lumbar disc removal was performed in Germany at the turn of the twentieth century. The first patient had a complete relief of pain but the surgeon misinterpreted the disc tissue as a benign tumor of cartilage. Harvey Cushing performed a laminectomy on a patient thought to have a disc protrusion compressing the cauda equina and causing weakness in the legs. Cushing did not find a disc and he concluded that the disc must have slipped back into place. Another American neurosurgeon Walter Dandy reported two cases with sciatica in which he found loose cartilaginous disc fragments in the spinal canal mimicking a spinal tumor. He felt the fragments were caused by trauma.

As noted in Chap. 4, Mixter and Barr in 1934 revolutionized our understanding of lumbar disc disease. Their first patient was a 28 years old man who presented with typical symptoms of sciatica with limited motion at the lumbosacral joint and a positive straight leg raising test on the affected side. Mixter and Barr performed an L2 to S1 laminectomy and removed an approximately 0.5 in. disc fragment from the spinal canal and the patient had a complete recovery from the sciatica. They compared the material recovered at surgery to disc tissue obtained from a postmortem specimen and concluded that the material was indeed a ruptured disc. With the publication of 19 cases in their 1934 article the diagnosis of a "ruptured disc" became generally accepted in the medical community. Other surgeons shortly thereafter reported large series of patients successfully undergoing discectomy and by the 1960s this was the most frequent operation performed by neurosurgeons and orthopedic surgeons in the United States.

Surgical techniques have made huge advances since the time of Horsley and Cushing so that minimally invasive microsurgeries (using a microscope) are now the standard at most major medical centers in the world. Sometimes, a protruded disc, bony overgrowth or even a small tumor can be removed with an endoscope so that post-operative healing is more rapid and the procedure can be done as an outpatient.

Surgery vs. Conservative Treatment for Disc Herniation

Given that in most cases, it is possible to document nerve decompression with MRI after surgery an equally important question is whether surgical decompression leads to better long-term outcome compared to spontaneous healing (i.e. conservative management). Just as with surgery, there are many cases of disc herniation with nerve compression documented on MRI that spontaneously resolve on follow-up MRI. It is still unclear in the long run whether surgery leads to a better outcome than spontaneous healing. The classic randomized controlled study comparing surgery and conservative care for acute disc herniation was published more than 30 years ago. It found that although patients who underwent surgery did better at 1 year follow-up, there was no difference in outcome between surgical and conservative care at 4 and 10 years follow-up. A more recent randomized controlled treatment trial in the Netherlands found similar results at 5 years follow-up but there were important caveats. By 6 months almost half of the conservatively treated patients required surgery because of severe persistent leg pain and disability. Therefore although conservative treatment of acute sciatica may give patients a reasonable chance of recovery without surgery such patients run the risk of eventually needing surgery and suffering with sciatica for months before the surgery.

Comparison of Different Surgical Techniques

Are newer microsurgical techniques any better than the traditional open laminectomy. Overall no difference has been found in outcomes or recurrences when comparing microdiscectomy versus open laminectomy. But since microdiscectomy surgery leads to a more rapid recovery with a shorter hospital stay it has largely replaced open discectomy surgery. Another important question is whether aggressive disc resection leads to better outcomes than removal of just the offending disc fragments so-called sequestrectomy. Although both procedures show comparable complications and repeat herniation rates sequestrectomy has a higher satisfaction rate so it is the procedure of choice.

As noted earlier, there is general agreement that most patients with low back pain and sciatica due to herniated discs get better without surgical treatment. On the other hand, there is also convincing evidence that patients with acute severe sciatica with mild or no back pain have a much more rapid resolution of symptoms after surgery than with conservative management. The results of surgery are much less impressive in patients with long standing back pain and sciatica. Microdiscectomy pioneer John McCulloch outlined eight basic principles that patients and physicians should understand when considering surgery for herniated discs (Table 6.1).

Table 6.1 What patients and physicians should know when considering back surgery for a herniated disk

| Herniated disks are common – lifetime prevalence of 1–2% |
| More than 90% get better without surgery |
| Only 2–4% of patients are candidates for surgery |
| MRI will identify herniated disks in 20–30% of asymptomatic people under the age of 60 years |
| Surgery improves short term outcome but probably not long term outcome |
| Surgery is rarely indicated before 6 weeks of symptoms but should not be delayed beyond 3–4 months |
| The disk will continue to degenerate with any form of treatment |
| Scar tissue will form making future surgery more difficult |

Modified from McCulloch JA. Focus issue on lumbar disc herniation: macro- and microdiscectomy. *Spine*. 1996;21:45S–56S

In the last 20 years a variety of percutaneous procedures have been developed to treat sciatica. The most common technique is to use an endoscope to visualize and enter the intervertebral foramen to remove osteoarthritic bony overgrowth, synovial cysts or herniated discs. Tiny rongeurs (heavy-duty forceps for removing small pieces of bone or tough tissue) and radiofrequency probes are passed through the endoscope to remove the offending tissue. Although large studies comparing endoscopy with traditional surgical methods are not available the two procedures seem to be comparable with success rates in the range of 60–70%. There is an extended learning curve for the surgeon to perform endoscopy effectively without complications and pain relief may be delayed compared to microsurgery operations. Endoscopic techniques have been used to remove tumors such as schwannomas near or in the intervertebral foramen but not intradural tumors involving the cauda equina. In these cases open visualization is important to avoid damage to nearby nerves and to obtain a good seal of the dura to prevent spinal fluid leakage.

Surgical Complications

One cannot consider surgery options without knowing potential complications. Surprisingly, one of the most common complications is operating at the wrong disc level or side. Herniated discs also can be missed or only partially removed even when the surgeon opens the proper location. These types of complications can be avoided with proper preoperative planning and training and with intraoperative imaging. Other important complications include infection, postoperative bleeding, nerve damage from positioning, and postoperative scarring. Between 5% and 15% of patients will have a recurrent herniation after disc surgery with the risk of recurrence decreasing with time after surgery.

Risk of Developing Chronic Postoperative Pain

Postoperative pain is one of the most frequent causes of chronic pain at a significant cost (monetary and social) to society. About a quarter of patients that suffer from chronic pain develop the chronic pain after surgery. Chronic pain can occur after any type of surgery although it is most frequent after operations lasting more than 3 h and operations producing a great deal of tissue damage. The highest rates of postoperative pain are associated with cardiothoracic and spine surgeries and with amputations.

Although chronic neuropathic pain can develop after any type of surgery it is more likely to develop when there are major nerves in the surgical field such as with sciatica surgery. To avoid intraoperative nerve injury the surgeon should perform a careful dissection, minimize inflammation and of course use minimally invasive techniques whenever possible. On average, patients undergoing surgery at high volume centers by experienced surgeons are less likely to develop postoperative chronic neuropathic pain suggesting that technique is important. Even when large nerves are not involved in the surgery, tissue retraction or cutting the skin or other tissues can damage sensory nerves and trigger chronic neuropathic pain.

Illustrative Cases Continued

Case 1

When Alfredo saw the orthopedic surgeon who specialized in back surgery, the surgeon showed him his MRI with the herniated disc and the surrounding inflammation. Because of these findings and his continued pain the surgeon recommended starting with an epidural steroid injection to treat the pain and also to confirm that the disc was causing his pain. When the surgeon explained how the injection was performed Alfredo expressed concern about pain during the procedure but he was reassured that he could be given a drug that would minimize the pain. The epidural injection went well and Alfredo had immediate improvement in his pain and after a week he was planning on returning to work but then the pain gradually returned. He had been slowly tapering off Vicodin but returned to taking two tablets every 6 h as the pain increased. When he returned to see the surgeon 3 weeks after the epidural injection (9 weeks after the onset of his sciatica) they decided that it was time for surgery. The surgeon told Alfredo that he could remove the disc fragment through a percutaneous endoscope so there would be only a tiny opening in the skin and the procedure could be done as an outpatient. He warned him that the pain can persist after surgery but it should then gradually subside. After regaining consciousness after the surgery Alfredo was told that the surgery went well and the disc fragment was successfully removed. He had to stay in the surgical recovery room for several hours until the effect of the general anesthetic resolved and his wife drove him home where he immediately went to bed. Alfredo was given a prescription for hydromorphone (Dilaudid) tablets for his post-operative pain and as the effect of the anesthesia subsided his pain increased and he initially took the hydromorphone 2 mg every 4 h but then increased to 4 mg every 4 h.

Comment

The decision regarding the timing of surgery for Alfredo's herniated disc presents a dilemma for patients and surgeons. Would Alfredo have fared better if surgery had been done earlier in the course of his sciatica? Since most patients get better with or without surgery initial conservative management is recommended but many patients will eventually require surgery and suffer from pain for week to months before undergoing surgery. Furthermore, waiting might increase the risk of a poor outcome from surgery. There is convincing evidence that the longer pain persists the greater the chance of developing central sensitization to pain. The picture is even more complicated in Alfredo's case because of his chronic use of opioids for pain control. These issues will be addressed in Chap. 7.

Case 2

Lamar saw the neurosurgeon about 6 weeks after his injury still complaining of pain radiating down the back of both legs that was markedly aggravated by any vigorous exercise. He wanted to return to competitive gymnastics but it was impossible for him to train. After reviewing his MRI the neurosurgeon indicated that he had two options; continue with symptomatic treatment of the pain and hopefully gradually returning to training when and if the pain improved or undergoing surgery to stabilize the spine and then returning to training after a prolonged period of rehab. Lamar chose surgery because he was tired of dealing with the pain and he wanted to return to gymnastics.

The neurosurgeon told Lamar that he recommended an open laminectomy procedure with decompression of the nerve roots and fusion of the L5 and S1 vertebra to prevent the slippage from recurring. He preferred the open procedure since it would allow good visualization of the nerve roots minimizing the risk of intraoperative injury. This would require a large skin incision and detachment of paravertebral muscles but he felt that it would offer the best chance for long-term recovery. The surgeon indicated that during the surgery he would first remove any bone that was compressing the spinal nerves and then fuse the L5 and S1 vertebrae using a bone graft and stabilizing rods attached to the bony pedicles with screws. He noted that probably the rods and screws would be left in place after healing but that in 5–10% of cases the hardware is later removed if it causes pain and discomfort. The main risks of the procedure were about a 1 in 1000 chance of spinal nerve injury or infection. Breakage of the hardware was extremely unlikely.

Comment

Although patients with low grade L5 S1 slippage (<50%) can recover without surgery Lamar chose surgery since he was frustrated with the chronic pain and he wanted to return to vigorous exercise and hopefully to gymnastics. An important question that is currently unanswered is whether minimally invasive endoscopic techniques are as good as traditional open techniques for decompressing spinal nerves and fusing the vertebrae for spondylolisthesis. Some preliminary studies suggest minimally invasive techniques may be as good as open techniques with a shorter hospital course with more rapid recovery but as in the case with other endoscopic procedures surgeon training and experience are critical and in some cases minimally invasive techniques may not be practical. A large controlled trial of open vs. minimally invasive surgery for spondylolisthesis has just begun in Europe so hopefully more definitive data will be available in several years.

Case 3

I saw the neurosurgeon a few days after my MRI studies were complete. Our neurology and neurosurgery clinics were next to each other so I arranged to see him after both of our clinics were over late in the afternoon. He began by telling me the story of his father, also a physician, who died after he saw several physician friends on an informal basis, never having had a proper examination to identify an obvious tumor. He then proceeded to perform a detailed neurological examination that took about 30 min. It felt eerie having just spent the afternoon performing neurological examinations myself. This was one of many strange experiences that I had as a physician patient.

We then looked at the MRI of my low back together and he agreed that the tumors were schwannomas and that the larger one was causing my sciatica. He would take the larger one out and we would just watch the smaller ones with follow up MRIs. He recommended a standard open laminectomy so the tumor could be removed while at the same time monitoring the function of the spinal nerve it was compressing. He felt it would be better to have a full exposure so the tumor could be completely removed with the best chance of saving the surrounding spinal nerves. He provided one piece of disturbing news that haunted me for the 2 weeks wait before the surgery could be scheduled. Since the tumor was inside the dura, the sac that encloses the spinal fluid (see Fig. 3.1), I would have to remain lying flat for 72 h after surgery to decrease the chance of a spinal fluid leak. By contrast patients that undergo laminectomy for removal of a degenerative disc or osteoarthritic bone can get up and walk to the bathroom within hours after the surgery since the dural sac is typically not opened.

The next thing I remember I'm awakening in the surgical recovery room, groggy but still alive. My throat was sore from the breathing tube placed during surgery so I preferred not to talk. I was informed that the surgery took longer than expected (about 4 h), but it went well and the preliminary pathology report indicated that the tumor was a schwannoma. After an hour or so, I was taken to my room and transferred to a regular hospital bed. My next big hurdle was the roll from side to side every hour or so because I could not lie on my back due to the stitches. I had to stay flat because of concerns for a spinal fluid leak; there was an IV in each arm and a catheter in my bladder. Each roll across was exquisitely painful and difficult to accomplish since there was nothing to hold onto and the various tubes became entangled in my body. I spent hours thinking about devices that could have made the process easier. A trapeze bar that moved from one side of the bed to the other or just hung down at the center would have been a simple solution. I couldn't imagine that others hadn't had the problem before me.

The nurses decided to order an air mattress that did ease the pressure on my side but made the roll from side to side even more difficult since I sunk into the air mattress and could not get traction for the roll. My solution was to take more pain medication. Initially, I tried to minimize the use of narcotics because I remembered that they made me nauseated when I used them after my shoulder surgery. But pain can trump just about any logical thinking so I had them start a hydromorphone (Dilaudid) self administering pump that allowed me to take as much as I needed to control the pain. This got me through the night but next morning I began to retch and was concerned that vomiting could lead to a spinal fluid leak. The Dilaudid pump was removed and I intermixed ibuprofen (Advil) and acetamenaphen (Tylenol) with occasional intravenous Dilaudid.

The 72 h lying flat seemed like 72 days. I didn't feel like eating and when I tried, it was difficult to swallow. Day and night seemed to blend together since I was so drowsy from the medications. When the 72 h were up, it was as though a heavy weight had been lifted from my chest. Although initially I was weak and light headed, I was able to walk on my own and there was a dramatic improvement in my spirits. Even more important that terrible night pain that kept me from sleeping was gone. The next morning I was discharged.

Comment

In my case the decision regarding the timing of surgery was easy since I couldn't live with the terrible pain that occurred every night and the tumor although benign would only continue to grow. The standard open procedure seemed appropriate because of the risk to the surrounding nerve roots in the cauda equina during the surgery. We did discuss the possibility of extending the laminectomy to a higher level to remove the other two pea sized tumors but my surgeon felt that the increased risk with a wider opening was not warranted since these tumors are very slow growing and probably (hopefully) they would not cause symptoms within my lifetime. My white coat did provide some "perks" such as easy access to specialists and moving to the head of the line for pre-op blood tests but once I entered the hospital and was given my plastic name band I was just like any other patient. I faced all of the usual problems that patients face such as dealing with post-operative pain and the apparent lack of planning with regard to my need to regularly turning from side to side in bed.

Suggested Additional Reading

Finger S. Origins of neuroscience. A history into brain function. New York: Oxford University Press; 2001.

Fulton JF. Harvey cushing. A biography. Springfield: Charles C Thomas; 1946.

McCulloch JA. Principles of microsurgery for lumbar disc disease. New York: Raven Press; 1989.
Reddi D, Curran N. Chronic pain after surgery: pathophysiology, risk factors and prevention. Postgrad Med J. 2014;90:222–7.
Weber H. Lumbar disc herniation. A controlled, prospective study with ten years of observation. Spine. 1983;8:131–40.

Chapter 7
Why Does Pain Persist in so Many Cases?

Two questions that patients with chronic pain frequently ask are: "Why me?" and "Why now?" Clearly some individuals are more vulnerable for developing chronic pain than others. A subset of all patients who undergo surgery of any kind develop chronic pain with the lowest rate (5–30%) for simple procedures such as hernia repair and C-sections, an intermediate rate (30–60%) for chest and heart surgery and the highest rate (50–85%) for surgeries involving major nerves such as surgery for sciatica. Between 25% and 50% of patients who develop acute sciatica will go on to develop chronic sciatica whether or not they have surgery. Why is there such a wide variation in whether or not a person develops chronic pain?

Early Thinking on Pain After Nerve Injury

Chronic pain after nerve injury was first described centuries ago mostly related to war injuries. The pioneer French surgeon Ambroise Paré described "phantom limb" pain in the sixteenth century and was a pioneer in the development of prosthetic limbs. Paré who progressed from being a barber–surgeon to the surgeon of four French kings, developed his skills in the many wars between Spain and France at the time. The invention of guns in the early sixteenth century led to an exponential increase in the number and severity of war wounds. Paré frowned on the common practice of using boiling oil and cauterization to sterilize wounds because it damaged healthy tissue and could lead to chronic pain. He simply cleansed the wounds of foreign debris to allow natural healing. Paré was one of the first to use a tight tourniquet to block pain signals in nerves originating from the wounded extremity and thereby reduce pain during amputation.

Paré was also one of the first surgeons to treat chronic pain by cutting the peripheral nerve supplying the painful area. He even considered cutting the offending nerve when Charles IX suffered intense pain in his arm after receiving a small pox vaccination. Fortunately for the king the pain gradually resolved without the need

© Springer International Publishing AG, part of Springer Nature 2019
R. W. Baloh, *Sciatica and Chronic Pain*,
https://doi.org/10.1007/978-3-319-93904-9_7

for surgery. An obvious problem with this approach is that large peripheral nerves in the arms and legs are made up of both sensory and motor components. Cutting the peripheral nerve causes loss of pain but also loss of all other sensations and paralysis of the muscles supplied by the nerve. Paradoxically, cutting a peripheral nerve can lead to chronic neuropathic pain that can be more bothersome than the original pain.

The American neurologist, Silas Weir Mitchell, was also known for his work on painful war injuries. Mitchell was stationed at the South Street Hospital in Philadelphia during the American Civil War, called the "Stump Hospital" by the soldiers. He noted that 95% of men experienced some feeling of the limb still being present after amputation. Most reported that the phantom limb felt shorter than the real limb and most complained of pain in the phantom limb. The soldiers were rarely comfortable with their stump and for years the stumps were tender and easily hurt and could suddenly become very painful. Some tried to protect the stump from any kind of stimulus since touch and even wind could trigger pain. Mitchell felt that the pain was caused by irritation of the nerves in the cut stump and he tried a range of treatments including burning the nerves in the stump and using a variety of drugs all with relatively little success. Some suffered so greatly that they begged for and received a second amputation higher up usually with no different outcome than the original amputation.

Mitchell along with wartime colleagues George Reed Morehouse and William Williams Keen published a classic text on pain and wartime injuries in 1864 about a year before Lee's surrender at Appomattox. The book provided detailed descriptions of the wide range of painful conditions associated with gun shot injuries. The most dramatic pain syndrome described in the book later became known as causalgia, combining the Greek words for heat and pain. The soldiers described the pain as "burning," "mustard red hot" or like a "red hot file rasping the skin". Mitchell and colleagues noted that the pain made the sufferer anxious and irritable and markedly interfered with sleep. The extremity became exquisitely sensitive to pain so that the slightest touch of a finger triggered extreme pain. The soldiers became fanatical about not letting anything near the extremity including exposure to air. Some found relief in moisture preferring to keep the hand constantly wet.

Mitchell felt that causalgia was caused by irritation of a nerve at the wound site somehow interfering with the blood circulation and nutrition of the affected limb. The pain was typically associated with secondary changes in the skin, muscles and joints in the area innervated by the damaged nerve. The skin became shiny, red and tight and the muscles and joints contracted. Hair fell out and the limb could be wet with constant sweating or excessively dry from lack of sweating. Mitchell and his colleagues tried a range of treatments for causalgia including counterirritants and injecting morphine into the painful site all with little benefit. Like the soldiers with phantom limb pain some soldiers with causalgia asked to have the affected limb amputated but even then the pain persisted.

The earliest evidence that tissue injury might cause a hypersensitivity to pain within the central nervous system came from clinical observations in patients. In the late nineteenth century the Scottish Neurologist, James MacKenzie speculated that an injury could cause hypersensitivity to pain by producing an "irritable focus" in the spinal cord from the barrage of pain signals coming from the injured tissue. A half century later, pain surgeon William Livingston at the University of Oregon suggested that afferent pain signals from injured tissue triggered an abnormal firing pattern in the spinal cord. He speculated that reverberating circuits were set up within interneurons in the dorsal horn of the spinal cord causing a spread of hyperactivity to other areas including the sympathetic ganglia. Activation of the sympathetic nervous system caused the vascular changes and a viscous cycle developed causing further hypersensitivity at the injured site. A few years later pain researchers James Hardy, Howard Wolff and Helen Goodell at Cornell University in New York performed a series of experiments on themselves and on volunteer patients demonstrating that hypersensitivity to pain develops at some distance from the site of nerve injury. Like Livingston they speculated that the injuries caused a state of hyperexcitability in the spinal cord by activating interneurons that amplify and spread the increased pain sensitivity to adjacent areas.

The Spinal Cord Pain Gate

The Canadian psychologist, Ronald Melzack and British physiologist, Patrick Wall introduced the notion of a pain "gate" in the spinal cord in their famous 1965 *Science* article "Pain Mechanisms: A New Theory". Their gate control theory proposed that small (unmyelinated or thinly myelinated) pain and temperature sensing fibers and large (heavily myelinated) touch, pressure and vibration sensing fibers carried information from the site of injury to the dorsal horn of the spinal cord where they activated two types of neurons, transmission neurons whose axons carry pain signals up to the brain and inhibitory interneurons whose axons feedback onto the transmission neurons to impede their activity (Fig. 7.1). Both the small and large sensory

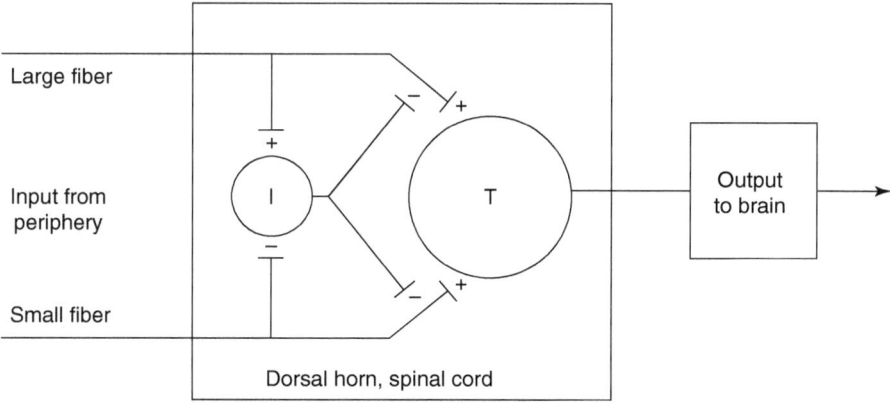

Fig. 7.1 Spinal cord pain gate as proposed by Melzac and Wall. Large fiber sensory input increases inhibition of pain transmission whereas small fiber sensory input decreases inhibition. I inhibitory interneuron, T transmission neuron

fibers excite transmission neurons but small fibers inhibit the inhibitory cells (allow-ing the transmission cells to fire) while large fibers excite the inhibitory neurons (decreasing the firing of transmission cells). In other words the inhibitory neurons act as a "gate" to control pain transmission in the dorsal horn of the spinal cord. The greater the large fiber (touch, pressure, vibration) activity relative to small fiber (pain and temperature) activity at the inhibitory cell, the less pain is felt. Melzack and Wall suggested that the pain gate could explain why touching or applying pres-sure or vibration to a painful extremity can ease the pain. It also provided a theoreti-cal foundation for the use of implanted devices for chronic electrical stimulation of peripheral nerves or the spinal cord for treating chronic neuropathic pain (see Chap. 8). Melzack and Wall also speculated that signals carried by the transmission neu-rons to the brain could, depending on the state of the brain, activate neurons that send signals back down the spinal cord to modulate the activity of the inhibitory cells (the "gate"). Thus they suggested an explanation for how the brain might influ-ence pain transmission in the spinal cord. More recently this brain pain control system that includes the prefrontal, cingulate and hippocampal cortices and the brainstem periaqueductal grey (PAG) and the rostroventromedial medulla (RVM) became known as the descending pain modulatory system (DPMS) (see Fig. 2.4).

In the early 1970s investigators in the United States and Sweden used radioac-tively labeled opioids like morphine to show that the brain has specific sites (recep-tors) that bind these drugs. More potent drugs were bound tighter than weaker drugs. Why would the brain have receptors for the product of a poppy plant? The answer came a few years later when researchers in Scotland the United States isolated opium like substances from the brains of normal pigs and calves. Opium and its derivatives just happen to be structurally similar to naturally occurring neurotrans-mitters in the brain. The first opioid neurotransmitter identified was called encepha-lin (from the Greek word for cerebrum) and the class of neurotransmitters called endorphins (combining endogenous and morphine). Numerous opioid receptors were subsequently identified. Opioid neurotransmitters and receptors are located throughout the brain and are involved in many functions but the highest concentra-tion of opioid transmitters and receptors is found in the DPMS particularly in the PAG region of the brainstem. Opioids block pain transmission in the spinal cord via the DPMS. They are also expressed in the respiratory and nausea and vomiting cen-ters in the brainstem; this explains why respiratory suppression and nausea and vom-iting are bothersome side effects associated with use of opioid drugs.

Role of the DPMS in Developing Chronic Pain

Studies of peripheral nerve injury in rodents suggest that endogenous opioids and the DPMS play an important role in whether or not chronic pain develops. In a rat model of sciatica, compression of a lumbosacral spinal nerve results in chronic neuropathic pain with hypersensitivity to pain in between 50% and 85% of animals depending on their genetic background. Injecting the local anesthetic, lidocaine, into the RVM, the key brainstem relay center of the DPMS, prevents the chronic pain from developing (see Fig. 2.4). The RVM contains inhibitory "off" and excitatory "on" neurons, that project to and control the "pain gate" in the dorsal horn of the spinal cord. When opioids are given systemically or injected into DPMS brain centers, RVM "off" neurons increase firing and "on" neurons decrease firing blocking pain transmission in the spinal cord.

Studies in neonatal and adolescent rats show that there is a critical period in development of the DPMS during which the descending opioid pathway through the RVM transitions from primarily facilitation to inhibition. This raises the interesting possibility that nerve injuries that occur early in life could alter the "set point" of the DPMS increasing the likelihood for developing chronic pain later in life. The change in the balance between excitatory and inhibitory influence of the DPMS on pain input that typically occurs in preadolescent animals is influenced by hormonal levels and is different in males and females.

DPMS and Placebo Effects

Major advances in our understanding of central pain control in humans came with the development of functional magnetic resonance imaging (fMRI) a technique that quantifies nerve activity in different brain centers in real time by measuring changes in glucose uptake and blood flow (see Chap. 5). The glucose uptake and blood flow to a brain center increases and decreases in proportion to the nerve cell activity in that center. Typically, a baseline measurement is made and then another measure is made after a painful stimulus is applied. By subtracting the baseline scan from the pain scan, areas with significant increase or decrease in nerve cell activity are identified as important for pain perception. Early studies with fMRI confirmed that humans share the same brain pain pathways as other primates. Normal humans show increased nerve cell firing in the lower brainstem, the thalamus, and throughout the cortical pain-related pathways after a painful stimulus is applied anywhere on the body.

Some of the most interesting work with fMRI is with regard to placebo drugs and analgesia. Remarkably, the same feedback pathways in the DPMS that are activated by opioid drugs are activated by placebo. Furthermore, high placebo responders show more activity in these areas than low responders during opioid analgesia. Since opioid receptor binding potential at baseline and after a painful stimulus varies markedly from individual to individual, it is likely that high placebo responders have a more efficient endogenous opioid system than low placebo responders. In other words, your ability to respond to placebo pain relief is directly related to the efficiency of your endogenous opioid system. It is also highly likely that other non-drug methods of analgesia such as meditation, acupuncture, and hypnosis work through this same endogenous opioid feedback system. Functional MRI studies have found that the subject's belief and expectation strongly influenced the degree of cortical activation and the degree of pain relief.

The Autonomic Nervous System and Chronic Pain

The concept of two different nervous systems, one in charge of voluntary behavior and the other in charge of vegetative processes dates back to the eighteenth century. In his famous book *Recherches physiologiques sur la vie and la mort* (Physiological researches upon life and death) published in 1800 the French anatomist and physiologist Marie François Xavier Bichat noted that vegetative functions such as circulation, intestinal absorption and glandular secretion can continue after brain death. He suggested that there were two lives, the animal life and the organic or vegetative life. After observing patients with severe brain injuries he noted that animal life which involved conscious and voluntary activities stopped while vegetative life which involved the activity of the deep internal organs such as the heart and intestines continued. He correlated this observation with his anatomical studies that showed that the deep internal organs received almost no cerebral nerves but many nerves from the ganglionic nervous system (a series of small independent "brains" in the chest cavity – the autonomic ganglia).

The next big breakthrough in understanding of the autonomic nervous system came in the late nineteenth century and early twentieth century from William Gaskell and John Newport Langley working in Cambridge, England. Gaskell studied the origin of the efferent (outgoing) component of spinal nerves and distinguished between somatic motor nerves from the spinal cord and splanchnic nerves from the ganglia system (Fig. 7.2). Somatic nerves caused contraction of skeletal muscles and the splanchnic nerves contraction of smooth muscles (the muscles in the walls of internal organs such as blood vessels and gut). Further he noted that

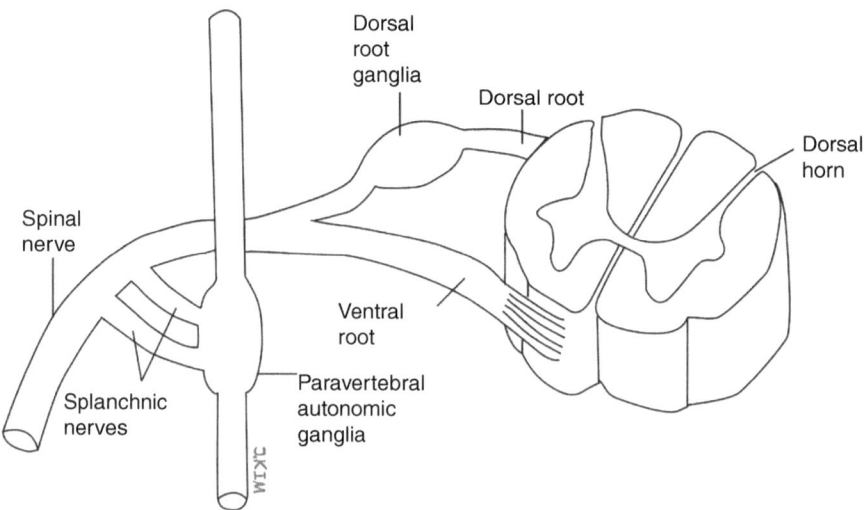

Fig. 7.2 Relationship between autonomic ganglia and sensory and motor roots of spinal nerves. Splanchnic nerves carry sensory and motor signals to and from the autonomic ganglia located along the vertebral column

there were two parts to the ganglia system: one part that supplied smooth muscles that contracted in the presence of adrenalin which he called the sympathetic system and another part that supplied smooth muscles that contracted in the presence of acetylcholine, later named the parasympathetic system by Langley who also introduced the term autonomic nervous system. Langley outlined the anatomical features of the preganglionic and post ganglionic fibers that made up the sympathetic and parasympathetic systems. He believed that the autonomic system was purely an efferent system without afferent nerve fibers and that there was no possibility of pain sensibility or reflex behavior at the level of the ganglia.

Others including the pioneering French physiologist Claude Bernard, felt that there must be afferent nerve fibers in the sympathetic nervous system just as they were in the somatic system. Bernard noted that he could cause pain in animals if he irritated the superior cervical ganglia of the sympathetic nervous system. In 1893 the English Neurologist, Henry Head suggested that when visceral and somatic afferent nerves enter the spinal cord at the same level, visceral pain may be perceived as a somatic pain at that level (so-called referred pain). For example, cardiac pain is referred to the left arm and kidney pain to the flank.

Like Bernard the French neurosurgeon, Rene Leriche, felt that there must be a specific sympathetic sensibility since patients reported severe pain if the sympathetic nerves or ganglia were inadvertently damaged during surgery. As an example of sympathetic pain he pointed to the intense pain (angina) that occurred in patients with cardiac ischemia. He argued that the cervical sympathetic ganglia must be a sensory-motor reflex center since he obtained good pain relief in patients with angina by ablating the inferior cervical ganglia. As with many other neurosurgeons of the time Leriche sharpened his skills during wartime where he treated many soldiers with nerve injuries including causalgia. Sympathectomy surgery (removing the sympathetic ganglia) sometimes relieved the terrible pain of causalgia when nothing else worked. Leriche popularized "pain surgery" in his book *La Chirurgie de la douleur* (Surgery of Pain) published in 1937 in which he summarized his experience with operating on the central and sympathetic nervous systems in patients with chronic pain. In the book he gave a good description of chronic neuropathic pain in which the pain is so overwhelming that the other symptoms are secondary.

Injuries to the sympathetic nervous system can cause pain but even more important activation of the sympathetic system can modulate pain and trigger secondary changes in metabolism of tissues in the area of the pain. Visceral afferent pain fibers run in peripheral nerves and splanchnic nerves to the sympathetic ganglia and then back to the spinal nerves to enter the spinal cord so injury to any of these structures can activate visceral pain fibers. These visceral afferents can be activated directly by compression or by the "inflammatory soup" surrounding the nerve injury. Increased firing of visceral pain fibers can trigger reflex sympathetic outflow through the connections in the paravertebral ganglia and spinal cord which in turn can cause increased blood flow, temperature changes and skin changes in the affected extremity. Release of noradrenalin from sympathetic fibers can stimulate immune cells and pain fibers that express adrenergic receptors. A viscous cycle can develop as activation of visceral afferents leads to reflex activation of the sympathetic system that in turn triggers inflammation and activation of both visceral and somatic pain afferent fibers. Pain activation of the sympathetic system may lead to a variety of secondary tissue changes including changes in temperature, circulation, swelling, changes in skin texture and color and local sweating. Pain signals reaching the limbic system can trigger hypothalamic outflow providing a generalized activation of the sympathetic system along with fear, anxiety and depression. This mechanism can cause panic reactions with racing of the heart, chest pressure and tightness and a smothering sensation. Many of these secondary symptoms are frightening and confusing and understanding how they occur can be helpful for breaking the viscous cycle aspects of the symptoms.

Neural Plasticity and Chronic Pain

A basic feature of all living organisms is the ability to adapt to their surroundings. Even single cell organisms can respond to noxious stimuli with evasive behavior. Animals with a nervous system modify behavioral responses by modifying the connectivity within the nervous system. In the late nineteenth century, the Russian physician and physiologist Ivan Petrovich Pavlov conducted a series of experiments that revolutionized our understanding of neuronal plasticity. Based on his simple observation that dogs in the laboratory would drool when they saw a lab coat Pavlov surmised that the dogs associated the lab coat with food because they always received food from someone wearing a lab coat. To prove his theory he developed a method to accurately measure saliva production and changed the "conditioning stimulus" from a lab coat to a loud noise, ringing a bell. If he rang a bell each time that food was presented after multiple trials the animals would automatically increase salivation when the bell rang even without food. This learning to associate the bell with salivation would dissipate with time after the training stopped but could be reinstated with a brief period of retraining. Pavlov also studied the animals' responses to a noxious stimulus such as a painful shock to the foot. Normally animals rapidly withdrew the extremity, the pupils dilated and the heart rate and breathing rate increased. If a benign stimulus such as a touch or a bell ring was presented immediately after the painful stimulus the animals had the same response to the benign stimulus as to the noxious stimulus as though the nervous system became hypersensitive to all stimuli. If the noxious stimulus was repeated multiple times the animals gradually decreased their response, a type of habituation. If the noxious stimulus was withdrawn for a period of time and then reintroduced the animal responded to it as with the initial exposure.

Pavlov, who was the first Russian to win the Nobel Prize, surmised that there must be changes in the brain associated with these different types of learning but knowledge regarding neuronal mechanisms was rudimentary at the time. In 1894, the Spanish anatomist Santiago Roman y Cajal, formulated the "neuronal theory" based on the idea that axons terminated next to the cell bodies and dendrites of other neurons and not in a latticed network as was generally accepted at the time. He speculated that the junctions (synapses) between the axon terminals and the cell bodies and dendrites were important for learning within the brain and that the connections between neurons could be reinforced by multiplication of the axonal terminal branches. Jerzy Kornorski, a Polish neuropsychologist who spent 2 years in Pavlov's laboratory, was the first to use the term plasticity to describe the changes that occurred in the brain with learning. He proposed that neuronal systems were plastic and could change permanently based on the number and combination of incoming action potentials. By the mid twentieth century two basic mechanisms were considered to explain learning within the nervous system: (1) changes in neuronal networks with branching of nerve terminals and (2) changes in the amount and type of transmitters and receptors at synapses.

Central Sensitization to Pain

Following peripheral nerve injury structural and chemical changes occur in central pain pathways that can persist long after the injury has resolved. Just as in the primary pain neurons secondary pain neurons in the spinal cord can show increased spontaneous firing rates, decreased thresholds for firing and increased response to incoming pain signals. Chronic inflow of peripheral pain signals into the dorsal horn can change protein expression in the secondary transmission neurons including the number and type of receptors. With peripheral nerve injuries growth factors released from axon terminals in the dorsal horn result in sprouting of thick myelinated afferent fibers that terminate deeper in the dorsal horn. These sprouting fibers gain access to partially denervated secondary pain neurons in the more superficial layers of the dorsal horn resulting in a cross talk between the sensory systems.

A basic feature of chronic neuropathic pain in the dorsal horn of the spinal cord and at pain relay stations in the brainstem and brain is an increase in excitatory transmission and a decrease in inhibitory feedback. With repetitive firing of peripheral pain fibers transmission neurons in the dorsal horn increase the number of action potentials generated per incoming action potential, a kind of "winding up" of the system. Further, repetitive winding up leads to long-term potentiation (LTP) with increases in the number of excitatory receptors expressed in transmission neurons. The time frame for winding up is minutes whereas it is days to months for LTP, time for new proteins to be synthesized. At the same time inhibitory feedback decreases after peripheral nerve injury with decreased expression of inhibitory opioid and serotonin receptors in the transmission neurons and interneurons.

Not only do primary pain neurons release chemicals into the dorsal horn but supporting glial cells also release chemicals after nerve injury that lead to enhancement of pain transmission. An important subgroup of glia, microglia, normally function in the central nervous system as white blood cells do in peripheral tissues. Shortly after a peripheral nerve injury microglia accumulate in the superficial layer of the dorsal horn within the termination zone of the injured nerve axons and release a wide variety of signaling molecules including many of the same cytokines that form the inflammatory soup associated with tissue injury. These molecules activate receptors on secondary neurons and enhance central neuronal sensitivity and persistent pain associated with nerve injury. Interestingly, microglia are not activated by inflammatory tissue injury but only with nerve injury. So there must be a signal generated by nerve injury unrelated to pain fiber firing that is specific for microglial activation.

Early neurologists and neurosurgeons were largely unimpressed with the role of the cerebral cortex in pain perception. In 1927 the English neurologist Gordon Holmes noted that he had never seen a patient develop a loss of pain sensitivity after a cortical lesion. By contrast patients with damage to the somatosensory cortex in the parietal lobe lose all touch sensation in the skin area projecting to the region of damage. Harvey Cushing was one of the first to electrically stimulate the somatosensory cortex in patients undergoing brain surgery under local anesthesia and although his patients reported sensations of touch they did not report pain. Yet, if the somatosensory cortex is stimulated in patients with chronic pain they experience pain. The chronic input of pain signals somehow changes the somatosensory cortex. For example, a patient with long standing sciatica will report pain when the leg area of the somatosensory cortex is stimulated. Furthermore, stimulating the nearby area that normally just receives input from the arm will also trigger pain in the leg. The chronic pain signals not only change the response of the leg area of the somatosensory cortex but also the neighboring arm area. The changes in central pain representation are even more remarkable after amputation of an extremity. Branching axons from nearby areas innervate the neurons that have lost their input from the amputated extremity.

Genes and Chronic Pain

A number of genetic mutations and variations have been associated with either decreased or increased sensitivity to pain. Mutations in the nerve growth factor (NGF) receptor gene, TrkA and in the sodium channel gene, Nav 1.7 are associated with congenital insensitivity to pain (mentioned in Chap. 1). Different kinds of genetic mutations in Nav 1.7 can lead to either a complete loss of pain sensitivity or hypersensitivity to pain with conditions called erythromelalgia and paroxysmal extreme pain disorder, both of which produce excruciating burning pain. Mutations in the sodium channel gene, Nav 1.8, cause hypersensitivity to pain and have been found in three percent of patients with painful neuropathy of unknown cause. Several different types of calcium channels are expressed in the dorsal horn and some appear to be selectively expressed in pain neurons. Animals with mutations in the genes for the N-type calcium channels Cav 2.2 and Cav 3.2 have reduced pain sensitivity after inflammation or nerve injury. A calcium channel blocker, ziconotide, when injected into the spinal fluid surrounding the spinal cord, is effective for treating intractable cancer pain (see Chap. 9). The antiseizure drugs gabapentin (Neurontin) and pregabalin (Lyrica) that are widely used to treat chronic neuropathic pain work by blocking a subunit of calcium channels that are upregulated after nerve injury (see Chap. 8).

A curious phenomena that was largely folklore until recently was the observation that red headed people were more sensitive to pain and less sensitive to anesthesia than people with other hair colors. Some surgeons were reluctant to operate on red heads because of their perceived decrease in pain threshold. To test whether these anecdotal observations were accurate investigators compared the effectiveness of the local anesthetic lidocaine in protecting against painful electrical stimulation of the skin in women with red hair and women with dark hair and found a significant decrease in pain tolerance in red heads. Since red hair is nearly always associated with mutations in the melanocortin-1 receptor gene (*MC1R*) this gene is likely important for pain transmission. Studies in mice support this observation and suggest that the MC1R gene effect on pain sensitivity may be female specific through mechanisms still to be worked out. About 3% of people in the world have red hair but as many as 15% of people in Scotland have red hair.

Clinicians have long been aware of a wide variation in individual responses to opioid drugs. Some patients require small doses whereas others require massive doses to obtain the same pain relief. Some patients have severe side effects while others have few side effects and some are easily addicted while other are resistant to addiction. Since these variations in the response to opioid drugs often run in families genetics likely play an important role.

Four nucleotide bases, adenine, cytosine, guanine and thymine form the backbone of DNA and carry the genetic code for protein production. All human beings share most of the same genetic code (what makes us human) but variations called single nucleotide polymorphisms (SNPs) occur about every 100–300 base pairs in the human genome and represent about 90% of human genetic variability. Close family members share more SNPs than more distant family members. Indeed checking a sampling of SNPs can determine heritage and how closely two individuals are related (testing that is now available through several internet sites). The effect of a SNP depends on whether or not it is in the coding region of a gene, which nucleotide is changed and where in the gene the change occurs. A common SNP in one of the opioid receptor genes, a change from adenine to guanine at position 118 (A118G), has been implicated in a wide variety of conditions including drug addiction, stress response and treatment response to opioid drugs. The A118G SNP is associated with a decreased pain threshold and a reduced response to opioid drugs in patients being treated for chronic pain. Interestingly, higher doses of opioid drugs required by patients with the A118G SNP do not produce increased respiratory depression so that these patients can tolerate higher doses. The A118G SNP is most common among Asians (40–50%), less common in Europeans (15–30%) and least common in African Americans and Hispanics (1–3%). Exactly how this single base change in the opioid receptor gene causes the change in pain threshold and pain response to opioids is still being worked out but it does illustrate the importance of slight genetic variations in determining drug response and suggests that in the future treating patients with pain may require knowledge about individual genetic variability before prescribing pain medication.

Are genetic or environmental factors more important for developing chronic pain? Clearly much of neuronal connectivity and function are determined by genetic expression during development. The number, location and connectivity of most neurons is genetically predetermined. Yet, the strength of the connectivity can be altered with experience so that even identical twins do not respond the same to different environmental stimuli. Heritability of chronic pain in identical twins is somewhere between 15% and 60% depending on the cause and severity of chronic pain. So the answer is genes and environment are probably about equally important in the development of chronic pain.

Priming of the Pump

There is convincing evidence from animal and human studies that early life injuries and stressors may play a role in later development of chronic pain. For example, neonatal chronic foot shock or maternal separation in rodents can lead to heightened pain sensitivity when the animals are fully developed. Similarly rodents will later develop pain hypersensitivity if they are exposed to repeated low level inflammatory injuries or if they are stressed with unpredictable loud sounds. Proposed mechanisms for this priming include: changes in the opioid DPMS, changes in nerve growth factor induced neuronal plasticity and changes in spinal microglia. Treatment with minocycline, an inhibitor of microglia activation, reduces priming in one rodent model.

To see if painful procedures performed in a neonatal ICU on preterm infants might cause long-term alterations in pain processing, researchers used fMRI to assess the response to a moderately painful heat stimulus in adolescents who had been in a preterm neonatal ICU compared with an age matched group who had not been in an ICU. They found that the adolescents who had been in a preterm neonatal ICU showed significantly greater activation of brain pain pathways than the controls and that the activation was pain-specific and not observed during non-painful warm stimulation. Furthermore, the adolescents who had been in a neonatal ICU tended to be more sensitive to the painful stimuli and didn't develop habituation as easily to the controls. Either the pain or the stressors of being in a preterm ICU lead to later development of hypersensitivity to pain.

In adult humans prior exposure to pain also appears to predispose to developing chronic neuropathic pain. Studies in young girls with episodic pain associated with menstruation throughout early adulthood found that they are more likely to develop central sensitization to pain than controls without menstrual pain. People with severe pain in an extremity prior to amputation are much more likely to develop phantom limb pain after amputation than people without limb pain prior to surgery. Similarly, intense pain prior to any surgery predisposes to developing post-operative chronic neuropathic pain. People who have intense pain with a herpes zoster infection (shingles) are more likely to develop chronic post-herpetic pain. Just as in animals there likely are a variety of mechanisms to explain these priming effects in humans including changes in the DPMS and spinal microglia and psychosocial factors such as fear and anxiety.

Age

In the rodent model of sciatic and chronic neuropathic pain, ligating a lumbosacral spinal nerve in infant rats causes sciatica and spinal hypersensitivity to pain similar to in adults but the hypersensitivity dissipates much more rapidly in the infant rats than in adults and it is more difficult to induce chronic neuropathic pain in infant rats. Similarly chronic neuropathic pain is unusual in children and adolescents probably related to age specific changes in brain pain pathways including the DPMS mentioned earlier.

Sleep and Chronic Pain

There is a tight interrelationship between sleep and chronic pain. The majority of patients with chronic pain report poor sleep. A viscous cycle often develops whereby sleep disturbance from chronic pain leads to psychosocial and behavioral factors that worsen the sleep disturbance. Poor sleep predicts the amount of attention paid to pain the next day that in turn predicts the quality of sleep the next night. Even in healthy volunteers sleep deprivation magnifies pain. Patients with chronic pain have abnormal sleep onset, sleep quality and the total amount of sleep and electroencephalographic (EEG) monitoring during sleep shows more light sleep with less slow wave deep sleep, less rapid eye movement (REM) sleep, and frequent sleep arousals. These are stages of sleep each with a different EEG profile.

In addition to the psychosocial aspects of sleep deprivation there are several molecular mechanisms that might explain the effects of sleep deprivation on chronic pain. Typically during deep sleep afferent sensory signals including pain signals are blocked at the level of the thalamus so that they do not reach higher cortical centers. Frequent arousals allows pain signals to be passed on to the brain emotional centers. Decrease in REM sleep leads to a decrease in brain serotonin levels that could alter the descending pain modulatory system (DPMS) allowing pain signals to pass the spinal cord "gate". Finally, sleep deprivation causes increased production of inflammatory cytokines related to pain and alters hormone and nerve growth factor pain signaling.

Depression and Chronic Pain

There is a bidirectional relationship between pain and depression: pain causes depression and depressed subjects are more likely to develop chronic pain than subjects without depression. Neuropathic pain in particular is associated with depression. About half of patients with chronic neuropathic pain also have depression. It is not hard to imagine why chronic pain causes depression for anyone who has experienced chronic pain. It is difficult to enjoy normally pleasurable activities when experiencing constant pain. One becomes preoccupied with the pain. Pain signals activate the emotional brain, the limbic system, which is the key brain area involved with depression. Functional MRI studies show that similar areas of the brain (mostly in the limbic system) are functionally abnormal in subjects with chronic neuropathic pain and in subjects with depression.

If you have had a prior bout of depression you are more than twice as likely to develop chronic pain. But why are patients with prior depression more likely to develop chronic pain? Genetic susceptibility is important for both chronic pain and depression and likely there are genetic variants that predispose to both chronic pain and depression. We are just learning about the neurological basis for depression and there are clear structural and chemical changes in the brains of patients with depression. Limbic structures critical for chronic pain lose volume as measured on MRI in patients with depression. The monoamine neurotransmitters noradrenalin, serotonin and dopamine play important roles in both pain and depression. All three neurotransmitter systems interact with the opioid DPMS that modulates pain transmission in the dorsal horn of the spinal cord. The hallmark of depression is a dysregulation of these neurotransmitters. As we will see in Chap. 8, drugs such as duloxetine and venlafaxine that increase brain norepinephrine and serotonin levels, treat both depression and chronic pain. Drugs and placebos that activate the opioid DPMS also treat both chronic pain and depression.

Fear Avoidance Behavior

In the mid-nineteenth century, Claude Bernard introduced the concept that body systems overall function to maintain a constant internal environment that he called the internal milieu. The body maintains the internal environment by a range of compensatory reactions designed to restore a state of equilibrium in response to changes in the environment. The American physiologist, Walter B. Cannon, expanded on Bernard's theory in the early twentieth century and in the process founded an entirely new field of study, neuroendocrinology. Initially working on digestive disorders Cannon noted that pain and anger interrupted gastric secretions and impaired digestion whereas happiness and satisfaction improved digestion. To study the phenomena, he applied normally painful electrical stimuli to anesthetized animals and noted increased secretion of adrenalin into the blood from the adrenal glands that was associated with increased breathing rate, dilation of the pupils, increased blood glucose, improved lung capacity and increased circulation to the heart, lungs, muscles and brain at the expense of the viscera. All of these effects could later be reproduced in the same animal by simply injecting adrenalin into the blood stream. Cannon explained these findings in evolutionary terms suggesting that these primitive reflexes served the purpose of "survival of the fittest". He coined the term "fight or flight" which were the only two options available between primitive prey and predator. Cannon felt that the adrenalin release from the adrenal glands was under control of the autonomic nervous system reflexively activated by the painful stimuli.

As suggested earlier in the chapter, the autonomic nervous system controls automatic body reflexes such as blood pressure, heart rate and respiration rate. The primary neurons for the autonomic system are located in the hypothalamus, part of the limbic pain system pathway. The hypothalamus is the key brain neuroendocrine center and pain has the potential to affect all body organs through activation of the limbic system and release of a wide range of hormones.

Since pain normally signals impending danger or harm it is not surprising that patients with pain might avoid activities such as exercise that can induce or exacerbate pain. While this may be an appropriate reaction to acute pain, fear-avoidance behavior can lead to increased disability with chronic neuropathic pain. Muscles become weak, joints become stiff and bones become thinner. Fear of pain may be a better predictor of chronic disability than the degree of pain itself. Fear of the long-term consequences of surgery predicts those who develop chronic postoperative pain. Understanding the viscous cycle nature of the fear/pain interrelationship can help break the cycle. Anxiety and neuroticism prone subjects are more likely to develop the viscous cycle of fear and pain. The fight or flight response leads to the release of adrenalin and other hormones that increase anxiety and pain. Anticipation and anxiety activate limbic pain centers on fMRI leading to heightened pain perception.

Living with Chronic Neuropathic Pain

As suggested earlier in this chapter, sleep is a key issue in dealing with chronic pain. If patients have a good night sleep they often will have a good day in dealing with pain. On the other hand, the worst days come after a bad night sleep. Sleeping pills on a regular basis is not the answer since they become less effective after a few weeks. Occasional use for a bad night leads to better results. Regular daily exercise is key to living with chronic pain. Exercise not only improves sleep but also helps relieve pain by releasing endogenous opioids and enhancing the DPMS.

Another area that requires constant effort is to avoid negative thinking. With a bad pain day it is natural to wander whether something new is happening. Even if patients are given a reasonable understanding of the mechanism of chronic pain it is common for them to wonder whether something changed or something new has happened. Catastrophising, always expecting the worst, increases the disability associated with chronic neuropathic pain. If one anticipates a catastrophic consequence of an activity such as exercise one will avoid the activity. Patients need constant reassurance that their activities are not causing the chronic pain.

There are good days and bad days and it is natural for the patient to try and identify something he or she did to cause the bad days. But much of the fluctuation is random noise. Rumination about what one did to aggravate the pain is counterproductive. The patient needs to develop a plan to deal with the pain and stick with it.

Illustrative Cases Continued

Case 1

About a week after surgery Alfredo was still taking hydromorphone 4 mg every 4 h when he began noticing that his leg was becoming very sensitive to any type of stimulation including just touching the leg. At night the touch of his bed covers triggered a burning pain not just in the area of the prior sciatica but over the entire leg. He tried increasing the dose of hydromorphone to 6 mg but if anything the sensitivity of his leg increased so that he was unable to sleep more than a few hours before awakening with pain.

Comment

Alfredo was developing the typical features of central sensitization to pain with: (1) increased sensitivity to noxious stimuli with spread of the sensitivity beyond the area of the original pain and (2) pain triggered by normally non-painful stimuli such as light touch (called allodynia). The picture was complicated by his increasing dose of opioids. Although patients often develop tolerance to opioids requiring increasing doses to maintain pain relief the changing pattern of the pain suggests the likelihood of opioid induced hyperalgesia (OIH). The mechanism of OIH is poorly understood but likely involves enhanced long-term potentiation (LTP) as occurs with other types of chronic neuropathic pain. A trial of tapering the opioids and drugs that block LTP should be considered (see Chap. 8).

Case 2

Immediately after surgery Lamar had a band of numbness beginning in the back of his right thigh, radiating down to the outside of his calf into the outside of his foot. His surgeon told him that the loss of sensation was in the distribution of the right S1 spinal nerve that was probably slightly damaged during the surgery. He reassured Lamar that this numbness should gradually improve with time. Lamar's pain was improved but he was instructed to avoid exercise for several weeks to allow his back to heal. At about 2 weeks after surgery Lamar began noticing a burning tingling sensation involving his entire right leg. The pain was aggravated by activity so he markedly curtailed his activities preferring to sit with his leg propped on a pillow. Then he began to notice generalized swelling and increased sweating in his right leg. In addition to the generalized burning pain he noted the knee and ankle joints were painful when he moved them. When examined, his right leg was swollen, darker in color and warmer than the left leg.

Comment

Lamar had developed typical features of causalgia in his right leg. In modern times the term, causalgia has been replaced by the term, complex regional pain syndrome (CRPS) to reflect the fact that the syndrome can result from nerve damage (CRPS type II) or occur spontaneously (CRPS type I). The hallmark of CRPS is chronic burning pain associated with autonomic nervous system dysfunction. Although CRPS is relatively rare after back surgery (about 1 per 1000 cases), back surgery is the most common cause of CRPS involving the lower extremities (accounting for about one third of all cases). As we will see in Chap. 8 a range of treatments have been used for this disabling disorder but no single treatment has been consistently effective.

Case 3

After returning home after my surgery it was great to sleep in my own bed again even though I couldn't sleep on my back because of pain from the surgical incision. I had a band of numbness down the outside of my right leg into the great toe and ball of the foot in the distribution of the L5 spinal root but this was a minor nuisance. A week later I started to walk on the treadmill at first very slow but gradually increasing the speed. The terrible pain that awakened me during the night prior to surgery was gone so I could sleep throughout the night. But as I began to taper the ibuprofen after a few weeks, pain returned, a burning pain deep in the buttock in the same general location as the pain I had had before surgery but in a wider area. My left leg and buttock became very sensitive to any kind of stimulation and at night I was constantly moving and removing the bed covers in an attempt to get comfortable. It took several days to partially regain control of the pain with ibuprofen 800 mg every 6 h. Then the problems with my stomach began again, pain and nausea. I was in a bind. I continued to have pain when I stopped taking the ibuprofen, but it was causing irritation of my stomach when I took it regularly and it wasn't working that well anyway. Prilosec cut down stomach acid and helped with the nausea, but not the stomach pains. I continued to have a constant, deep, burning sensation in the buttock with occasional sharp stabbing pain down the leg similar to the pain I had prior to surgery. The stabbing pain although intense at times, was not nearly as bothersome as the constant deep burning pain.

Comment

Of all surgeries for sciatica, removal of a schwannoma from a lumbosacral spinal nerve has the highest risk for developing chronic neuropathic pain (>50%). Presumably it is impossible to remove the tumor without damaging the nerve. The band of numbness in the L5 spinal nerve distribution clearly indicated damage to the L5 spinal nerve. Interestingly I had some of the same type of pain I experienced before surgery but also developed a new more generalized pain along with allodynia.

Suggested Additional Reading

Denk F, McMahon SB, Tracey I. Pain vulnerability: a neurobiological perspective. Nat Neurosci. 2014;17(2):192–200.
Eccleston C. Role of psychology in pain management. Br J Anesth. 2001;87:144–52.
Nathan PW. Pain and nociception in the clinical context. Philos Trans R Soc Lond. 1985;B308:219–26.
Reddi D, Curran N. Chronic pain after surgery: pathophysiology, risk factors and prevention. Postgrad Med J. 2014;90:222–7.
Usdin TB, Dimitrov EL. The effects of extended pain on behavior: recent progress. Neuroscientist. 2016;22:521–33.

Chapter 8
Treatment of Chronic Neuropathic Pain

Some drugs used to treat new onset sciatica are also effective for treating chronic sciatica but there can be problems with long-term usage. For example, anti-inflammatory COX inhibitors such as the NSAIDs are helpful for treating chronic sciatica associated with inflammation such as due to osteoarthritis. With chronic high doses, however, irritation and bleeding in the gastrointestinal tract are common. Toward the end of the twentieth century pharmaceutical companies rushed to develop COX inhibitors with fewer side effects. In 1999 Merck and Co. received FDA approval for the selective COX-2 inhibitor, rofecoxib (Vioxx) and in 2001, Searle and Co. obtained FDA approval for celecoxib (Celebrex). Both companies marketed the drugs as the new wonder drugs for treating chronic arthritic pain.

But problems arose. With longer use, Vioxx was found to cause an increased risk of heart attacks particularly in older men. This was unexpected since earlier trials did not identify the risk. The maker, Merck & Co., was inundated with lawsuits from patients who had heart attacks while on Vioxx. In one widely reported trial, a lawyer won a multimillion dollar lawsuit using a new powerful technique, dubbed "CSI: Power Point". He teamed up with a computer entrepreneur who specialized in making power point presentations using a story-telling structure rather than the usual bullets, graphs, and charts. The lawyer used 253 slides in his opening argument and the jury awarded the wife $253 million, a million per slide. Vioxx was removed from the market in 2007. Celebrex remains on the market even though it probably has the same risk for heart attacks as Vioxx.

The story of Vioxx illustrates a problem the pharmaceutical industry faces when developing new drugs for treating chronic pain. Selective COX-2 inhibitors are examples of a wave of new drugs being designed to target specific proteins important in the initiation and transmission of pain (see Chap. 9). There were already many drugs on the market that inhibit COX-2 such as aspirin and the NSAIDs but these drugs have multiple other actions including inhibiting COX-1 which protects the lining of the stomach and intestines. The logic was that a selective inhibitor of COX-2 would be safer with fewer side effects. But it is impossible to predict the long-term effects of any new drug until it has been used for many years. The costs

© Springer International Publishing AG, part of Springer Nature 2019
R. W. Baloh, *Sciatica and Chronic Pain*,
https://doi.org/10.1007/978-3-319-93904-9_8

of discovering and testing a new drug for treating chronic pain can be astronomical only to find out later that there are unexpected side effects. As we will see later in this Chapter there are ways around this dilemma but these are not necessarily in the best interest of patients with pain.

In situations where a peripheral nerve has been compressed and damaged, an ideal drug would be one that stabilizes the damaged nerve and prevents the development of central sensitization to pain. Drugs such as antiepileptic and antidepressant drugs that block ion channels and neurotransmitters that are important for pain transmission are such drugs but all of them have multiple effects on the central nervous system. There have been multiple treatment trials demonstrating efficacy of antiepileptic and antidepressant drugs for treating chronic neuropathic pain associated with diabetic neuropathy and post-herpetic neuralgia. By comparison, there have been only a few controlled treatment trials in patients with chronic sciatica and the results have not been impressive. Of course chronic sciatica has multiple causes and some causes may be more responsive to treatment than other causes.

Ion Channels and Chronic Pain

The first hint of how nerve transmission might occur came at the end of the eighteenth century when an Italian biologist, Luigi Galvani, serendipitously observed that he could make a frog's leg twitch by stimulating it with a pulse of electricity. He proposed that nerves and muscles generated electrical currents and that the muscle twitches he observed were caused by electricity not "animal spirits". As strange as it may seem now, this was a revolutionary idea since at the time people believed that living organisms were governed by fundamentally different principles than inanimate objects. Herman von Helmholtz, mentioned previously in Chap. 2, was the first to measure the speed of the action current as it moved down the frog's nerve to activate a muscle. A remarkable technical feat for the time, Helmholtz had to measure the fraction of a second it took for the action current to move between two electrodes on the nerve. The action current was surprisingly slow (about 30 m/s) particularly when one considers that electricity moves along a copper wire with a speed of about 300,000,000 m/s. Obviously the nerve was not acting as a simple conductor of electricity like a wire.

In 1870, the German physiologist, Julius Bernstein, first suggested how electric currents in nerves (which he called action potentials) could be generated. He proposed that nerve fibers are normally electrically polarized, with the external surface of the membrane positive in relation to the internal one, and that the action potential was a self-propagated depolarization of the membrane. It was almost a century later that Bernstein's theory was conclusively proven by English physiologists, Alan Loyd Hodgkin and Andrew Huxley who received the Nobel Prize in Medicine and Physiology in 1963 for their model that showed how ion channels in the nerve fiber membrane open and close as an action potential moves along the nerve.

Ions are atoms or molecules in which the total number of electrons is not equal to the total number of protons so that they have a net positive or negative electrical charge. For example table salt is a compound of positively charged sodium ions (Na+) and negatively charged chloride ions (Cl⁻) forming the neutral salt, NaCl. Salt dissolves in water because water molecules are bipolar (a positive charge on one end and a negative charge on the other end) and can bind to both the Na+ and Cl⁻ ions. The human body is mostly water so ions are present in all tissues including nerves. The membranes of nerve fibers have selective ion channels, proteins that cross the membrane forming a pore, that allow just one type of ion to pass, for example positively charged sodium ions. When the axon is at rest, the channels are mostly shut. As an action potential comes along from the nerve cell body, the change in voltage opens sodium channels and positively charged sodium ions flow into the nerve fiber rapidly changing the membrane potential from negative to positive (Fig. 8.1). The sodium channels then abruptly close and potassium channels open briefly allowing positively charged potassium ions inside the fiber to flow out rapidly returning the membrane potential to the baseline negative value. In between action potentials, other ion channel proteins (not sensitive to voltage) pump sodium

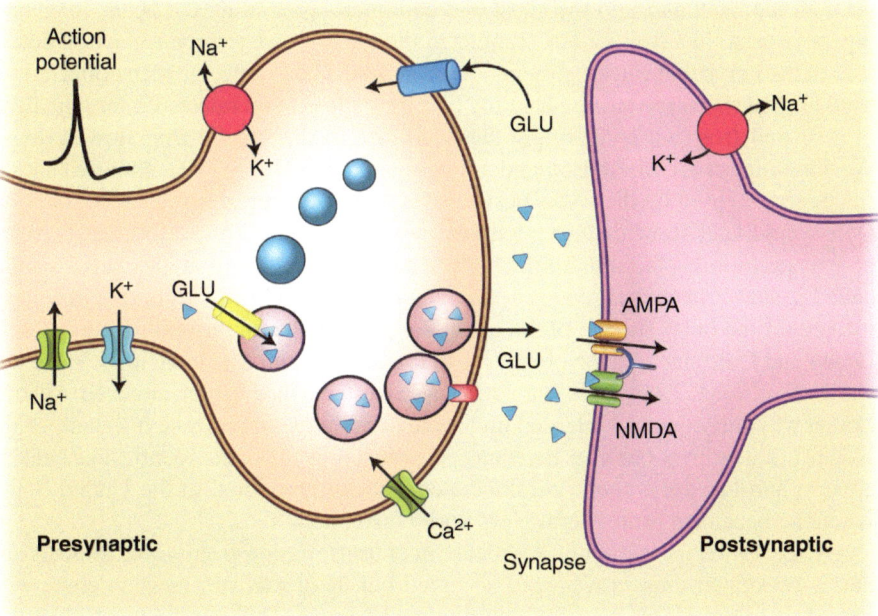

Fig. 8.1 Ion channels and synaptic transmission. The action potential moves along the nerve as Na⁺ and K⁺ channels open and close. When the action potential reaches the synapse it opens voltage gated Ca⁺⁺ channels that trigger the release of neurotransmitter, in this case the excitatory neurotransmitter, glutamate. The glutamate activates receptors in the post-synaptic membrane (AMPA and NMDA receptors) triggering an action potential and altering the number of receptors expressed in the post-synaptic membrane

out and potassium back in maintaining the status quo (a high concentration of potassium ions inside the axon and a high concentration of sodium ions outside the axon). After nerve injury, the density of ion channels increases in the damaged nerve fibers and the channels have different pharmacologic and depolarization characteristics. This explains why many current drugs that block ion channels (e.g. seizure drugs and antidepressant drugs) are useful for treating chronic neuropathic pain.

Brain Neurotransmitters and Chronic Pain

When the action potential reaches the axon terminal how does the signal cross the gap called a synapse, between the axon terminal and the neuron it contacts? Initial opinion was that the action potential, moving down the axon, jumped across the synapse like a spark and triggered an action potential in the next neuron. The first hint that a chemical might be released into the synapse by the axon terminal came in the 1920s when a German physiologist, Otto Loewi, working in Austria showed that the vagus nerve terminals in the heart released a chemical that slowed the heart rate. The vagus nerve, the tenth cranial nerve, runs from the base of the brain down through the neck and into the chest and abdomen innervating the heart, lungs and digestive tract. In a frog, Loewi stimulated the vagus nerve to produce action potentials in the nerve that caused slowing of the animal's heart rate. He then collected the fluid around the nerve terminals in the first frog's heart and injected it into the heart of a second frog and surprisingly the heart rate of the second frog slowed down. Working independently in England, a pharmacologist Henry Dale, showed that the substance released by the vagus nerve was a simple chemical, called acetylcholine. Dale would later show that acetylcholine was also released by motor neuron axons to activate muscles throughout the body. The basic idea was that the acetylcholine, called a neurotransmitter, crossed the synapse and bound to specialized receptors located on the outer surface of the target cell membrane, in this case a muscle cell. Loewi and Dale shared the Nobel Prize in Physiology and Medicine in 1936 for this work. Two years later Loewi, a Jew, was arrested when Hitler annexed Austria. Loewi was subsequently released under the conditions that he take his share of the Nobel prize from a bank in Sweden and transfer it to a Nazi-controlled bank in Austria and leave the country immediately. Loewi emigrated to the United States where he became a professor at New York University.

By the 1950s the notion of neurochemical transmission from nerve to heart and nerve to skeletal muscle was well accepted but there was still heated debate with regard to transmission between neurons in the brain. Those in favor of electrical transmission called "sparkers" led by the Australian neurophysiologist, John Eccles, argued that transmission between neurons occurred too fast to be mediated by a chemical. Whereas, those in favor of chemical transmission led by Henry Dale, called "soupers" argued that chemicals like acetylcholine could mediate rapid neurotransmission. As evidence for chemical transmission became more compelling, Eccles suggested that there might be two phases of neurotransmission, a rapid phase due to electrical transmission and a delayed slower phase due to chemical transmission. But it was soon shown that there was no need for electrical transmission. Acetylcholine rapidly diffused across the synapse and bound to a protein receptor in the muscle cell membrane causing the muscle to contract. The receptor had an acetylcholine binding site on the surface and an ion channel that crossed the cell membrane. When the acetylcholine bound to its site on the protein receptor it opened the ion channel pore which in turn triggered a muscle contraction.

After a period of brooding for losing the battle to the "soupers", Eccles became an enthusiastic champion for chemical neurotransmission. He made the important discovery that there is both excitatory and inhibitory synaptic chemical transmission in the brain. Excitatory transmitters decrease the membrane potential of target neurons while inhibitory transmitters increase the potential (making it harder for them to fire off). The balance of excitatory and inhibitory input determine whether or not an action potential occurs in the target neuron. Later work has shown that the main excitatory transmitter in the brain is the amino acid, glutamate and the main inhibitory transmitter is the amino acid, gabba-aminobutyric acid (GABA). When the action potential reaches the axon terminal it opens voltage gated calcium channels allowing an influx of calcium ions (Fig. 8.1). This causes a series of molecular steps leading to the release of small packets of neurotransmitter, called synaptic vesicles. These tiny vesicles filled with neurotransmitter fuse with the surface membrane releasing their neurotransmitter contents into the synapse. Multiple different receptors have been identified on the target cell membrane. One class of receptors, like the actylcholine receptor, are coupled with ion channels while another class of receptors activate second messengers inside of the target neuron that can alter the cells metabolism or enter the nucleus and activate genes for new protein production. Therefore some neurotransmitters can change the type and density of synaptic receptors on the target neuron over time. The diversity of information that can be transmitted across a synapse with chemical transmitters and receptors is several orders of magnitude greater than the information that could be transmitted with a simple electrical transmission.

Glutamate

Second order pain transmission neurons and interneurons express several different glutamate receptors but the initial rapid response is mediated by the postsynaptic AMPA receptors, which are transmitter activated ion channels (ionotropic). Binding of glutamate by the AMPA receptors causes an influx of positively charged ions that triggers an action potential in the target neurons (Fig. 8.1). Another glutamate receptor that is also ionotropic, the N-methyl-D-aspartate (NMDA) receptor, is normally quiescent but with increased firing of primary pain fibers after injury the AMPA receptors generate a strong depolarization of the target neurons causing the ion channels in the NMDA receptors to open, allowing more calcium to enter the postsynaptic neuron. The influx of calcium acts as a second messenger causing a cascade of changes in the postsynaptic neuron causing long-term potentiation (LTP). The calcium activates a protein enzyme called a kinase that increases synaptic strength and also signals for additional AMPA receptors to be assembled and inserted in the postsynaptic membrane. As noted in Chap. 6, LTP in postsynaptic neurons in the dorsal horn of the spinal cord is a major cause of hypersensitivity to pain after nerve injury. LTP is also critical for memory storage in the hippocampus, the memory center of the brain located deep within the temporal lobe. In the hippocampus, AMPA and NMDA receptors act as coincidence detectors, the presynaptic neuron must be active and release glutamate and the postsynaptic AMPA receptors must bind glutamate and depolarize the neuron. Only then will the NMDA receptors become active and trigger LTP causing a memory to be stored.

As we will see in Chap. 9, drugs that block excitatory glutamine transmission by binding to AMPA or NMDA receptors are promising treatments for chronic pain by preventing the development of central sensitization to pain after nerve injury. However, since excitatory neurotransmission occurs throughout the brain including the memory centers in the hippocampus these drugs have potentially bothersome side effects. For example, ketamine, a potent blocker of NMDA receptors produces a trance-like state along with pain relief, sedation and memory loss beginning about 5 min after injection lasting about 25 min. When ketamine was introduced in 1962, it seemed ideal for minor surgical procedures but later significant side effects on wearing off were identified including hallucinations, elevated blood pressure and muscle tremors. It has largely been replaced by midazolam and propofol as noted in Chap. 6. More recently, ketamine in smaller doses has been found to be effective for treating a range of refractory chronic pain conditions including chronic neuropathic pain, phantom limb pain, and causalgia (now called chronic regional pain syndrome – CRPS type II). In one small study, ketamine induced coma for 5 days in patients with refractory chronic pain lead to significant improvement in the chronic pain. This suggests the intriguing possibility that a complete shut down of pain pathways for a few days may "break the cycle" of chronic pain.

Gabba-Aminobutyric Acid (GABA)

The inhibitory neurotransmitter GABA is released by interneurons throughout the central pain pathways including the inhibitory "gate" neurons in the dorsal horn of the spinal cord. Drugs that mimic GABA, so-called GABA agonists, decrease pain transmission but also decrease overall brain activity. Barbiturates derived from barbituric acid were the first class of GABA agonist drugs. Phenobarbital (Luminal), the most commonly used drug in the class, was introduced as a seizure drug by Bayer in 1912 and by the mid twentieth century the broad range of psychoactive features of the drug became evident. Addictions and deaths due to overdose soon followed. In the latter part of the twentieth century barbiturates were largely replaced by a newer class of GABA agonists, benzodiazapines, which produce sedation with much less risk of overdose death. The benzodiazapines diazepam (Valium) and lorazepam (Ativan) are the most commonly prescribed drugs for anxiety and muscle relaxation and often these drugs are prescribed along with pain medications to treat chronic neuropathic pain. High doses are typically required for pain control, however, and as with the AMPA and NMDA blockers sedation and memory loss are bothersome side effects. Development of tolerance and dependency is also a problem. Midazolam, mentioned in Chap. 6 for its use with short medical procedures, is a benzodiazepine.

Opioids

As noted in Chap. 7, the descending pain modulatory system (DPMS) is a powerful central pain network that modulates pain transmission in the spinal cord and brain via the endogenous opioid system. All of the cortical and subcortical components have a strong input to and from the rostroventralmedial medulla (RVM) and the RVM projects down the spinal cord to the dorsal horn to control pain signals entering the spinal cord (see Fig. 2.4). This bidirectional central pain control system can alleviate pain when it is important for survival but it can also be responsible for maintaining chronic pain.

Although opioids are the most potent activator of the descending pain modulatory system (DPMS) surprisingly they are not very effective for treating chronic neuropathic pain such as chronic sciatica. This may be in part because opioid receptors are down regulated after nerve injury decreasing opioid inhibition via the DPMS. Not only are opioids not very good for treating chronic neuropathic pain, in some cases they may actually worsen chronic pain producing so-called opioid-induced hyperalgesia (OIH). With this condition, patients receiving opioids for treating chronic pain become more sensitive to pain (see Chap. 7).

Some of the weaker opioids such as tramadol also inhibit the reuptake of serotonin and noradrenalin further enhancing descending inhibition of pain (discussed below). But none of the opioid drugs are specific for pain control since there are opioid receptors throughout the central nervous system. Another major problem is tolerance and addiction. With the long term use necessary for chronic pain, more and more drug is required to obtain the same pain relief and physical dependency can develop. Use of opioids for treatment of back pain and sciatica is a major cause of the current epidemic of opioid addiction in the United States.

Noradrenalin

The locus coeruleus (LC), located in the high brainstem, is the main noradrenalin nucleus in the brain. The LC sends axons that release noradrenalin throughout the brain and plays a major role in arousal, attention and pain perception. There are projections to the amygdala and hypothalamus of the limbic system that trigger fear and anxiety associated with pain and threat including activation of the autonomic nervous system. Increased activity in LC is associated with anxiety and panic attacks and there is a strong association between chronic pain and chronic anxiety. Noradrenalin neuron projections to the dorsal horn of the spinal cord inhibit pain transmission by activating presynaptic noradrenalin receptors on the terminals of excitatory interneurons. Overall drugs that increase noradrenalin neurotransmission decrease pain transmission and are effective in controlling chronic pain.

Serotonin

Serotonin containing neurons are present throughout the brainstem with the highest concentration in the raphe nuclei located at the back of the brainstem near the midline. Projections to the limbic system are prominent and alterations in serotonin levels in the limbic system are associated with mood disorders such a depression. Serotonin is clearly involved in pain control but its role is complicated and it can inhibit or facilitate pain transmission. In rodent animal models injecting serotonin into the spinal fluid attenuates pain transmission at the dorsal horn in normal animals but has relatively little effect on chronic neuropathic pain. Serotonin clearly interacts with the DPMS since the opioid blocker naloxone attenuates the analgesic effects of injecting serotonin into the spinal fluid and serotonin blockers attenuate the effect of injecting morphine into the spinal fluid. However, serotonin also enhances the release of substance P that increases pain transmission in the dorsal horn. The picture is further complicated by the fact that a variety of serotonin receptors are expressed in transmission neurons and in both inhibitory and excitatory interneurons in the dorsal horn and serotonin can lead to increased expression of pain receptors in primary pain neurons such as TRPV1, the receptor sensitive to the chemical capsaicin found in chili peppers (see Chap. 2). As a general rule, drugs that increase serotonin levels decrease pain transmission but serotonin may play multiple potentially conflicting roles in pain perception depending on which neurons and which receptors are activated.

Dopamine

In 1954 James Olds and Peter Milner working at McGill University in Canada published their classical paper entitled "Positive reinforcement produced by electrical stimulation of septal area and other regions of rat brain." They reported that when electrodes were placed in the forebrains of rats, the rats would self stimulate these places regularly for long periods of time by pressing a bar that triggered the electrical stimulation even at the exclusion of other activities including eating. These areas in the brain that include the prefrontal and hippocampal cortex and several subcortical nuclei became known as the motivational/reward network and dopamine was shown to be a key neurotransmitter within the network.

The response to pain is highly dependent on activity in the motivational/reward circuitry and there is considerable overlap in the dopamine projections to these cortical and subcortical regions and between the reward network and the DPMS. Opioids modulate the dopamine signals defining different aspects of reward such as bliss, thrill and craving. The level of expression of dopamine receptors in the network determines ones ability to feel pleasure and pain. Dysfunction in the motivation/reward dopamine network is associated with a variety of clinical syndromes including mood disorders, neuropsychiatric disorders and chronic pain. Furthermore baseline activity in the neuronal centers of the network effects the magnitude of opioid induced analgesia via the DPMS.

Summary

A wide variety of neurotransmitters are involved in pain transmission. As a general rule, drugs that block glutamate transmission and drugs that enhance GABA, opioid, noradrenalin, serotonin and dopamine transmission decrease pain perception. The effect is more prominent for chronic pain than for acute pain. However, there are exceptions to this general rule particularly with regard to serotonin and dopamine and all of these neurotransmitters play multiple potentially conflicting roles in pain perception depending on which neurons and which receptors are activated. Considering the widespread distribution of these neurotransmitters and their receptors in the brain and spinal cord the fact that drugs that modulate the level of these neurotransmitters have troubling side effects is not surprising.

Antiepileptic Drugs

Antiepileptic drugs have been used to treat chronic neuropathic pain as far back as the early 1940s when phenytoin (Dilantin) was found to be effective for treating trigeminal neuralgia, a disorder characterized by sudden paroxysms of pain on one side of the face. Subsequently, carbamazepine and the newer drugs oxcarbazepine and lamotrigine have been used to treat trigeminal neuralgia and a range of other chronic neuropathic pain conditions including post-herpetic neuralgia, diabetic neuropathy and chronic sciatica. Effectiveness varies with different conditions and in different studies but can reach as high as 70%. These antiepileptic drugs work at least in part by blocking sodium channels thereby decreasing neuronal excitability. All of them are associated with serious side effects including Stevens-Johnson syndrome and idiosyncratic blood dyscrasias such as aplastic anemia and agraulocytosis but side effects are less common with oxcarbazepine and lamotrigine than with phenytoin and carbamazepine. These drugs have important interactions with many other drugs so physicians must be aware of these interactions before prescribing the drugs.

Currently the two most popular antiepileptic drugs for treating chronic neuropathic pain are the gabapentinoids, gabapentin (Neurontin) and pregabalin (Lyrica) (Table 8.1). Although initially introduced as antiepileptic drugs early studies on a range of seizure disorders with these drugs were not very promising. But then pregabalin was tried in patients with neuropathic pain caused by herpes zoster infections (shingles) and good results were reported. Double blind placebo controlled studies showed that pregabalin and gabapentin were significantly better than placebo in controlling chronic neuropathic pain. The mechanism of action is not completely clear but as noted in Chap. 7, gabapentinoids block a subunit of calcium channels expressed at the synaptic junction of pain fibers entering the spinal cord. The result is a decrease in excitatory transmission and a decrease in pain signals to the brain. Gabapentinoids also activate descending noradrenergic inhibitory pathways further blocking pain transmission at the level of the spinal cord. Although gabapentin and pregabalin have similar mechanisms of action, pregabalin is absorbed more rapidly than gabapentin and pregabalin absorption increases proportionately with increasing dose whereas gabapentin exhibits absorption saturation so that blood concentrations do not increase proportionally to increasing dose. Gabapentinoids are excreted in the kidneys and their effects last about 6–8 h. The main side effects are somnolence, weight gain, dizziness and rarely swelling of the extremities. Overall the gabapentinoids have no documented long-term toxicity or major drug interactions. Gabapentinoids may increase the risk of birth defects if taken in the first trimester of pregnancy so these drugs should be used with great caution in women who are or plan to become pregnant. Like with opioids, gabapentinoid abuse has become a big problem in the United States with approximately 1.5% of the general population abusing gabapentinoids. As high as two thirds of people that abuse opioids also abuse gabapentinoids. Many of these people were started on both medications for chronic back pain and sciatica.

Table 8.1 Pain medications commonly used for chronic sciatica

Class	Drug	Dosage[a] (as needed)	Main side effects
Tricyclic amines	Amitriptyline (Elavil)	25–150 mg at night	Drowsiness, constipation, weight gain
	Nortriptyline (Pamelor)	25–150 mg at night	Insomnia, constipation, weight gain
Selective serotonin and noradrenalin reuptake inhibitors	Venlafaxine (Effexor)	25–75 MG every 12 h	Sexual dysfunction, decreased appetite, constipation
	Duloxetine (Cymbalta)	30–120 mg per day	Nausea, sleepiness, constipation
Gabapentinoids	Gabapentin (Neurontin)	300–1200 mg every 8 h	Sleepiness, swelling, weight gain
	Pregabalin (Lyrica)	75–300 mg every 12 h	Sleepiness, swelling, weight gain

[a]Start with lowest dose and use the lowest effective dose

Antidepressant Drugs

Another major class of drugs used for treating chronic neuropathic pain is antidepressant drugs. The most widely used antidepressants for treating neuropathic pain are the tricyclic amines: amitriptyline, imipramine, and nortriptyline among others. These drugs are sometimes called "dirty" drugs since they have multiple modes of action. They increase serotonin and noradrenaline by blocking reuptake and they block sodium and calcium channels all potentially leading to decreased pain transmission. Overall, the different tricyclic amines have been about equally effective in clinical trials for neuropathic pain and all have bothersome side effects including sedation, weight gain, dizziness, constipation, urinary retention and sexual dysfunction. These drugs should be used with caution in patients with coronary artery disease, heart arrhythmias, known seizures, urinary retention, and glaucoma. A big problem with the tricyclic amines is potential drug interactions. They should not be used with other drugs that elevate brain serotonin and noradrenalin levels such as the selective serotonin and noradrenalin reuptake inhibitors and tramadol and they should be used with caution in patients taking NSAIDs and warfarin (can increase the risk of bleeding).

Another class of antidepressant drugs used to treat chronic neuropathic pain is the combined selective serotonin and noradrenaline reuptake inhibitors (SSNRIs). These drugs block the re-uptake of serotonin and norepinephrine at neuronal synapses leading to increased activation of the receptors of these two important neurotransmitters in the pain pathways. Since serotonin and norepinephrine provide excitatory input to the inhibitory interneurons in the dorsal horn of the spinal cord, SSNRIs help close the "gate" to pain signals arriving at the dorsal horn. Of course there are serotonin and noradrenaline receptors throughout the brain and other pain pathways may also be involved. Studies show that relief of neuropathic pain with SSNRIs occurs within hours of starting the drugs while the antidepressant effect of the drugs typically takes weeks so pain relief and depression relief are probably different effects of the drugs. Of the SSNRIs only venlafaxine and duloxetine have been studied and found to be effective in controlled treatment trials for chronic neuropathic pain. The main side effects include somnolence, constipation, nausea, dizziness, dry mouth, increased sweating and headache. Combined SSRIs and SNRIs should be used with great caution in patients with high blood pressure or in patients taking other drugs that increase serotonin including tricyclic amines and tramadol. They are contraindicated in patients with severe liver or kidney impairment.

Implanted Spinal Fluid Pumps

Injecting medications directly into the spinal fluid surrounding the spinal cord and spinal nerves can markedly increase the potency with less side effect risk. For example, opioids injected into the spinal fluid are about 1000 times as potent as oral opioids with less chance of addiction. But repeatedly placing a needle into the spinal fluid is not without risk and discomfort. So for treating chronic pain, surgically implantable drug reservoirs that pump precise doses of medication into the spinal fluid have been developed and once in place they can be easily and safely refilled with a needle and programmed for different doses. Of course, one must be extremely careful with dosing because of the increased potency of drugs directly injected into the spinal fluid. Some drugs, such as small peptides, can only be administered in the spinal fluid since they would be digested if given orally and do not cross the blood brain barrier if given intravenously (for example ziconotide discussed in Chap. 9).

Nerve and Spinal Cord Stimulation

Electrical stimulation of nerves or the spinal cord is another common technique used for treating chronic pain particularly neuropathic pain. As discussed in Chap. 7, the "gate" theory of Melzack and Wall proposed that activating large diameter sensory nerves that carry touch and vibration sensation excite inhibitory interneurons in the dorsal horn of the spinal cord blocking small fiber pain signals (see Fig. 7.1). Based on this premise, surgeons implanted plate electrodes over the dorsal columns at the back of the spinal cord where large fiber sensory nerves reside. The electrodes were connected to an electrical pulse stimulator that the patient could control. In these early trials a laminectomy was required to gain access to the spinal cord and the electrical stimulators were large and cumbersome but many patients reported good results. Over time it was found that tiny electrode arrays implanted via a percutaneous needle worked just as well as the large plate electrodes and these electrode arrays could be placed in the epidural space outside the dura or near spinal nerves entering the dura often with equally good results. What exactly the electrical stimulation was doing to stop pain transmission was not entirely clear but animal experiments suggest that the electrical current affects both spinal cord and brain pain centers.

Typically the procedure is performed in two steps. First a temporary electrode is implanted through a large needle and the electrode is connected to an electrical stimulator. The patient should feel tingling in the region of the pain if the electrode is in the proper location. The stimulator sends electrical pulses of different duration and amplitude to the electrodes to achieve the best pain control. During the trial period, that can last a few days to a few weeks, different pulse durations and amplitudes are tried and pain relief and functional activities are monitored with the goal of obtaining at least 50% relief of pain. If the trial is successful the electric pulse stimulator is implanted under the skin under local anesthesia where it can be programmed for the best results.

To date nerve and spinal cord electrical stimulation has proved most helpful for treating chronic radicular pain such as chronic sciatica. It has been particularly effective for treating so-called failed back surgery syndrome (FBSS), where patients have undergone multiple surgeries for sciatica but continue to have chronic pain.

About half of patients with FBBS obtain good pain relief with spinal cord electrical stimulation. Electrical stimulation for pain control is not without risks and complications, however. About a third of people will have some type of complication although most are minor. The most common complication is migration of the implanted electrode so that it no longer stimulates the correct area. This typically occurs within the first few days of implantation if it occurs. Not surprisingly, percutaneous electrodes are more likely to migrate than electrodes surgically implanted. Serious complications such as damage to a spinal nerve or the spinal cord by the percutaneous needle or bleeding into the space outside the dura occurs in only one to two percent of patients. Infection requiring a course of antibiotics occurs in up to 5% of people.

Ablation of Pain Pathways

As noted in Chap. 7, the notion that cutting a peripheral nerve supplying a painful area can relieve the pain dates back as far as the sixteenth century. As our knowledge of the anatomy of pain pathways advanced in the early twentieth century, a wide range of ablative procedures were developed to block pain signals at different levels within the peripheral and central nervous system. After an initial wave of enthusiasm for ablative procedures it became clear that there were significant complications and long-term results were disappointing. The basic notion that ablating a pain pathway can cure chronic neuropathic pain was rightfully questioned. Further, with the discovery of medications for treating chronic pain, the risk associated with ablative procedures was difficult to justify. However, as imaging and surgical techniques dramatically improved in the late twentieth century there was a renewed interest in the use of ablative procedures for treating chronic neuropathic pain. Needles and endoscopes can be more accurately guided so that selective ablation can be achieved with minimal risk to surrounding tissue. Due to the problems with current medications described earlier in this chapter, pain management centers are increasingly returning toward a procedural based approach. The problem is we have very little information on the long-term effectiveness of these procedures for treating chronic sciatica.

Peripheral Ablative Procedures

Cutting a peripheral nerve such as the sciatic nerve to treat chronic pain is not an option for obvious reasons. However, selectively cutting of the sensory root (rhizotomy) or ablating the dorsal root ganglia of a damaged spinal nerve can block pain signals without impairing muscle function. Loss of pain, temperature and touch sensation in the distribution of a single spinal nerve is usually a minor nuisance since there is overlap in the sensory distribution of nearby spinal nerves. The dorsal root ganglia can be ablated by injecting chemicals such as phenol or alcohol (with a local anesthetic) or by hot or cold probes or radiofrequency probes introduced through a needle guided by fluoroscopy. Although these procedures have been effective in treating some types of chronic neuropathic pain such as trigeminal neuralgia and post-zoster pain, the results in patients with chronic sciatica have been disappointing. Furthermore, the sensory roots and dorsal root ganglia of the spinal nerves that form the sciatic nerve are difficult to reach because of surrounding bone and specialists who perform these procedures require extensive training and must have a good understanding of the spine and nerve anatomy.

Although surgery and chemical ablation of the sympathetic ganglia have been used for almost a century to treat chronic pain we still don't completely understand the relationship between the sympathetic nervous system and chronic pain. It remains unclear whether it has a direct or indirect role in generating pain but the sympathetic nervous system is clearly involved in secondary features such as swelling and temperature changes in the affected extremity. As noted in Chap. 7, surgeons initially reported excellent results for treating the disabling symptoms of causalgia (CRPS II) but with long-term follow up the benefits were less impressive. The lumbar sympathetic ganglia lie along side the lumbar vertebra so they are relatively easy to access either with surgery or a needle. Recent studies using chemical ablation of the lumbar sympathetic ganglia have reported a success rate of 30–50% for chronic sciatica. Initial injection of a local anesthetic can produce a reversible ablation to help decide whether or not to produce a permanent ablation.

Central Ablative Procedures

In the early decades of the twentieth century investigators identified the pain pathways to the brain in animals using a variety of techniques including tracking degenerating axons after cutting the axons near the neurons of origin (Wallerian degeneration) (see Fig. 2.2). Postmortem examinations in patients with small lesions in the spinal cord and brain provided key information on defining the pain pathways in humans. An American neurologist, William Gibson Spiller, probably published the most convincing clinical pathological correlation with regard to the localization of the pain and temperature pathways in the spinal cord in 1905. A young man with tuberculosis developed a remarkably selective loss of pain and temperature sensitivity his left leg. Autopsy revealed a tiny, localized area of infection (a tuberculoma) in the right anterolateral column of the spinal cord. Based on this observation and published studies in animals (see Chap. 2), Spiller convinced a neurosurgical colleague, Edward Martin, to cut the anterolateral quadrants of the spinal cord in a man with severe chronic pain in his legs. The results of the surgery published in the Journal of the American Medical Association in 1911 reported that the patient had a great relief of the pain below the level of the surgery but still required a small regular dose of morphine. This technique was shortly followed by procedures that cut the midline of the spinal cord to interrupt the pain signals crossing to the opposite side (commissurotomy) and procedures that ablated pain pathways in the brain such as in the thalamus (thalamotomy) and the cingular cortex (cingulotomy) (see Fig. 2.4). As in the case with ablative procedures of the peripheral pain pathways these central ablative procedures were initially reported to have excellent results in treating chronic pain but with time they fell out of favor because there were major complications such as bleeding into the brain and the effects were limited in duration. With the development of modern stereotactic surgical procedures the focal ablations can be achieved with more precision and less risk but they are still only used as a last resort in patients who have failed all other forms of therapy. For example, recent studies of medial thalamotomy and anterior cingulotomy for treating refractory chronic pain found initial response rates in the range of 50% with up to 1% having serious complications.

Problems with Current Treatments for Neuropathic Pain

The problem with current medications used for treating chronic neuropathic pain is that they do not have a selective effect on pain pathways. Most have actions on nerve cells throughout the brain and spinal cord many of which are unwanted. The feeling of "dullness" that patients report while taking pregabalin is probably due to blocking of neurotransmitters in the hippocampus, the brain structure critical for registering memories. The nausea and indigestion with duloxetine is likely due to serotonin effects on the gut and on the nausea centers in the brain stem.

Why can't the pharmaceutical companies develop a drug that is selective for the pain pathways? It is possible but there are many obstacles. There are subtle differences between membrane proteins expressed in different locations so targeting proteins that are just expressed in peripheral and central pain pathways could be a strategy for a "magic bullet" drug that would shut off pain signals but have minimal side effects on other parts of the brain. Blocking such proteins in animal models of peripheral nerve damage alleviates some types of pain but it is unclear whether these drugs will be useful for patients with chronic neuropathic pain.

Ah but there's the rub. It costs pharmaceutical companies hundreds of millions of dollars to develop a new drug and take it through the clinical trials that are required to get approval from the FDA. Part of the process is to show that the new drug is effective and safe. And then there is always the possibility that after going through the tedious process set up by the FDA and the drug is approved some unexpected side effect will be identified either in the late stages of clinical trials or after the drug is on the market. A perfect example is the COX 2 inhibitor rofecoxib (VIOXX) as discussed earlier in this Chapter.

Pharmaceutical companies may have found a way around the FDA maze for introducing a new drug. They take an old drug that was previously introduced for some other condition (e.g. pregabalin, duloxetine) and test it against placebo for relieving chronic neuropathic pain. The beauty is that they don't have to show that the drug is as good or better than other drugs currently used for neuropathic pain just that it is better than placebo. They don't have to establish dosage and safety since this has already been done. They can put all of the money into marketing it as the new wonder drug for neuropathic pain.

In recent times there is a trend toward the greater use of procedures for treating chronic pain. This trend is in part due to the fact that medications aren't very effective and that technology advances have made the procedures easier and safer to perform. The fact that our current medical system rewards procedures at a much higher monetary rate than traditional medical examinations and treatments no doubt also plays a role. But we have very few long-term studies on the effectiveness of different procedures for treating chronic neuropathic pain and almost none using placebo controls. Short-term response does not predict long-term response and long-term risks and complications are largely unknown.

Case Illustrations Continued

Case 1

When Alfredo returned to the orthopedic surgeon a month after surgery he reported that his leg pain continued despite taking hydromorphone 6 mg every 4 h. There was a deep burning pain with occasional sharp shooting pains down the leg similar the pain he experience before surgery. His leg continued to be very sensitive to any type of stimulation even the light touch of his bed covers. The surgeon told him that he was concerned about his continued use of hydromorphone and that it might be actually making his pain worse. He recommended that Alfredo gradually lower the dose of hydromorphone and gave him a prescription for gabapentin (Neurontin) starting with 300 mg a day and gradually working up to 300 mg every 6 h over a few weeks as he tapered the hydromorphone. Alfredo noted definite improvement in his pain after starting the gabapentin and the initial drowsiness became less as he adapted to the new medication but any attempt to decrease the hydromorphone made him very uncomfortable so he continued on the prior dose. It was approaching 2 months post surgery and he did not feel that he could return to work. He called his surgeon who recommended a referral to the pain management clinic.

When Alfredo was seen in the pain management center they also raised concerns about his continued use of hydromorphone but suggested a trial epidural injection of steroids for pain relief and as a diagnostic test to see if inflammation of the spinal nerve was contributing to his continued pain. He had had an epidural injection prior to surgery that was successful so he agreed to the procedure. They gave him refills for the gabapentin and hydromorphone but the plan was to begin tapering the hydrocodone after the epidural injection and eventually stop the medication. His response to the second epidural injection was not as clear as after the initial injection but Alfredo did feel that there was some improvement in his leg pain. As the clinic staff began decreasing the amount of hydromorphone in his prescriptions Alfredo began replacing the hydromorphone with morphine obtained from a local dealer.

Comment

Alfredo's tragic story is being played out in communities throughout the United States. Patients are given opioids for treating back pain and sciatica and they become addicted and move on to street drugs that are readily available. Most patients are given a prescription for opioids on leaving the hospital after back surgery often with refills that last for weeks. As many as two thirds of people in the United States addicted to opioids also abuse gabapentinoids prescribed for chronic pain. With regard to managing his chronic sciatica beginning a gabapentinioid and referral to a chronic pain clinic would be a common approach. As noted earlier in this chapter, pain management centers are becoming more and more procedural oriented.

Case 2

Lamar's surgeon explained to him that he developed a rare pain condition (chronic regional pain syndrome, CRPS) that can occur after major back surgery and that paradoxically the pain is made worse by lack of movement and exercise. He arranged for Lamar to begin a physical therapy program and prescribed nortriptyline, a tricyclic antidepressant medication, used for treating chronic pain. He emphasized that Lamar must move the joints in his leg even though it was painful and that he could take ibuprofen on an as needed basis in addition to the nortriptyline. Lamar dreaded the physical therapy sessions because when the therapist moved his joints he experienced severe pain even though after the sessions there was improvement of the pain. The swelling in his leg improved as well but after several weeks of physical therapy Lamar was becoming frustrated since he could not exercise and it was still painful to walk and carry on normal activities such as returning to classes. When he was reevaluated a month later, his surgeon recommended a lumbar sympathectomy on the right side because there was still some residual swelling and increased sweating in the right leg. The surgeon felt that this along with continued physical therapy would lead to gradual recovery. After his lumbar sympathectomy, Lamar did gradually improve and after another month of physical therapy he was able to return to a regular exercise routine although he gave up his gymnastic career because he and his family did not want to risk the possibility of another injury to his spine.

Comment

Tricyclic amines are probably the most common drugs used for treating chronic neuropathic pain including chronic sciatica. Side effects can be a problem particularly sedation and anticholinergic effects such as dryness of the mucous membranes, urinary retention and constipation. Nortriptyline has less sedating and less anticholinergic effects than the other commonly used tricyclic amines. The role of sympathectomy in treating causalgia (complex regional pain syndrome type II) remains controversial but there is a general agreement that physical therapy with range of motion exercises is key to long-term recovery. With lack of activity, joints become stiff and bones become thinner and patients can become invalids.

Case 3

My neurosurgeon suggested I try pregabalin for my chronic sciatica since he previously had good success with the drug. The average effective dose for neuropathic pain is 150 mg twice a day but you have to build up to that level slowly. I began with 50 mg capsules first once a day and then twice a day and I noticed that I was drowsy throughout the day but I assumed that I would adapt to the drug. As I increased the dose to 75 mg twice a day, it was impossible to stay awake through the day and so I began taking it mostly at night. At least pregabalin allowed me to sleep better at night. At 2 months after surgery I was taking pregabalin 150 mg at night (the maximum I could tolerate) and ibuprofen 400 mg every 6 h but the pain continued. My stomach was constantly upset. I didn't think things could get any worse so I decided to taper off the pregabalin over several days. When I was finally off the pregabalin the pain was even worse than before. At night I would constantly be putting on covers and taking them off, sweating and then chilled. One night I didn't sleep at all not even for a few minutes. The next day at work was hell.

I had to find another drug to replace the pregabalin. After discussing the matter with a neurological colleague who specializes in pain management we decided to try an antidepressant drug in the SSNRI class, duloxetine (Cymbalta). She felt duloxetine had fewer side effects than the tricyclic amines, particularly the sedation and constipation. The usual dose is 30–60 mg, long release capsules so you only need to take it once a day. I started duloxetine 30 mg in the evening and within hours I noted improvement in the hot sensation over my thigh. The next day I was encouraged. The pain was noticeably less. I did notice some increase in my chronic indigestion that I attributed to the ibuprofen so I planned to taper the ibuprofen after a few days on duloxetine. By day three on duloxetine my encouragement turned to despair. My gut was hyperactive and I was so nauseated that I didn't feel like eating. I faced another dilemma. Was it the duloxetine or the ibuprofen?

I decided that my only course was to stop both duloxetine and ibuprofen and give my gut a rest. At that point I actually thought the pain was preferable to the nausea. My solution was Celebrex, the selective COX 2 inhibitor twice a day and extra strength Tylenol 2 capsules as needed. Neither of these drugs have significant gastrointestinal side effects. At night I used 150 mg pregabalin for sleep but not every night so that tolerance was less likely to develop. With this regimen I was able to function but the deep burning buttock pain continued and I constantly had to get up and walk around after sitting for any length of time.

Comment

In my case the drugs used to treat chronic sciatica were effective but side effects limited their use. Pregabalin caused sedation and a continuous "dopey" feeling and duloxetine caused nausea and gastrointestinal hypermotility. Interestingly, pregabalin is a reasonably good sleeping pill when used on an occasional basis. Why did my pain become more pronounced after stopping pregabalin? Pregabalin blocks a subunit of a calcium channel that is critical for release of excitatory neurotransmitter throughout the brain and spinal cord. Nerve cells respond by increasing the production of the calcium channels in an attempt to overcome the pharmacological block. You require more and more medication to maintain the same benefit over time (called tolerance). This is a slow process that occurs over days to weeks since it requires activation of genes, synthesis of new proteins and transport of the proteins to the cell membrane. After stopping pregabalin there was an excess of calcium channel subunits and an increased release of neurotransmitters in the pain pathways leading to hypersensitivity. Duloxetine blocks the reuptake of serotonin and noradrenalin at neural synapses leading to increased levels of these ubiquitous neurotransmitters. There are more serotonin receptors in the gut than in the brain so it is not surprising that duloxetine causes gastrointestinal hypermobility.

Over time I gradually learned to live with chronic sciatica. I learned to expect occasional bad days and overall I found that the less pain medication I took the better I did in the long run. I also found that regular exercise was a key to living with the chronic pain. Sometimes there was a paradoxical increase in pain after vigorous exercise but I found that overall I did much better with a daily exercise routine.

Suggested Additional Reading

Dworkin RH, O'connor AB, Backonja M, et al. Pharmacologic management of neuropathic pain: evidence-based recommendations. Pain. 2007;132:237–51.

Khoromi S, Cui L, Nackers I, et al. Morphine, nortriptyline and their combination vs. placebo in patients with chronic lumbar root pain. Pain. 2007;130:66–75.

Kremer M, Salvat E, Muller A. Antidepressants and gabapentinoids in neuropathic pain: mechanistic insights. Neuroscience. 2016;338:183–206.

Smith HS, Argoff CE, Kaur M, Nagaraja H. Gabapentinoids and other anticonvulsants. In: Toth C, Moulin DE, editors. The management of neuropathic pain. New York: Cambridge University Press; 2013. p. 225–39.

Chapter 9
Promising New Treatments for Chronic Pain

There is general agreement among researchers, clinicians and patients that we need better treatments for chronic neuropathic pain. With the rapid advances in our understanding of genetics and molecular biology in the last 25 years there is renewed enthusiasm that better treatments can be developed. Considering the complexity of pain transmission at the molecular level described earlier in this book, not surprisingly, there are a large number of potential targets for the development of new drugs. It is not the goal of this chapter to provide a complete list of potential new drugs for treating chronic pain but rather to provide examples of the process of new drug development and of several promising new drugs (Table 9.1).

Table 9.1 Potential targets of new treatments of chronic pain

Target	Mechanism	Example
Nerve growth factor (NGF) signaling	Block NGF components of chronic pain	Tanazumab, monoclonal antibody binds NGF and prevents pain cascade
Voltage gated ion channels	Block overexpressed Na^+ and Ca^{++} channels	Ziconotide, conotoxin derived peptide that blocks N-type Ca^{++} channels
Transient receptor potentials (TRPs)	Block TRPs in primary pain neurons	GRC17356, small molecule that blocks TRPA1 receptors
Opioid receptors	Enhance descending pain modulatory system (DPMS)	PZM21, selective μ-opioid receptor agonist
Cannabinoid receptors	Enhance endogenous opioid transmission	Sativex, mucosal spray combining THC and CBD
Glutamate receptors	Block central sensitization to pain	Traxoprodil, selective NMDA receptor blocker
Gamma-aminobutyric acid (GABA) receptors	Enhance inhibition in pain pathways	L-838,417, selective agonist of α_2 and α_3 $GABA_A$ receptors
Noradrenalin receptors	Enhance inhibition in pain pathways	Clonidine, a selective noradrenalin α_2 receptor agonist
Dopamine receptors	Activate motivation/reward network	Pramipexole, dopamine D_3 receptor agonist

© Springer International Publishing AG, part of Springer Nature 2019
R. W. Baloh, *Sciatica and Chronic Pain*,
https://doi.org/10.1007/978-3-319-93904-9_9

Prevention

The notion that chronic pain might be prevented by vigorously treating acute pain dates back more than a century. The American surgeon, George Washington Crile, published a paper in the English journal *Lancet* in 1913 in which he suggested that post operative pain could be lessened by using a local anesthetic in addition to general anesthesia to prevent the barrage of pain signals that occurred during surgery from entering the central nervous system. Crile served as a military surgeon during the Spanish American war in Puerto Rico and later in France during World War I and he was impressed with how the soldier's emotional state prior to surgery affected the outcome. Extreme pain and fear prior to surgery predisposed to developing pain after surgery. To improve the outcomes of surgery he used a variety of psychological techniques to alleviate fear and vigorously treated pain including anaesthetizing the operative region with the local anesthetic cocaine for up to several days before operating. Crile was one of the first to use blood transfusions and he developed several unique surgical instruments. He who was born and raised in Ohio and was one of the founding members of the Cleveland Clinic.

As our understanding of the role of tissue and nerve injury in producing central sensitization and chronic pain became clearer in the twentieth century the idea of vigorously treating acute pain to prevent chronic pain became popular. Animal studies showed that sensitization to pain that typically occurred after nerve injury could be prevented by an anesthetic block of the nerve input to the spinal cord prior to the injury. The amount of morphine needed to prevent the development of central sensitization to pain was an order of magnitude less than the amount needed to reverse the sensitization once it was established. Surgeons first began to use local anesthetics to block the spinal cord sensory input prior to amputating a limb. There are several variables that need to be investigated further such as the duration and type of pretreatment but most agree that some form of pain control before and during amputation surgery decreases the likelihood of developing chronic pain after surgery.

As noted in Chap. 6, chronic postoperative pain is a major source of morbidity even with minor surgeries such as tonsillectomy and hernia repair. A large number of recent clinical trials suggest that pre and perioperative treatment of pain can help prevent the central sensitization effects of the surgery. The severity of postoperative pain can be reduced and the amount of postoperative pain medications required is lessened. Perioperative nonsteroidal anti-inflammatory drugs (NSAIDs), opioids and local anesthetics can reduce the postoperative pain intensity and postoperative request for pain medications for a wide range of operations. Post operative incision pain is reduced by preoperative subcutaneous and intramuscular injection of local anesthetics. The reduced postoperative pain and the reduced postoperative pain medication required lasts much longer than the duration of the pre and perioperative agents administered. Whether pretreatment with drugs used to treat chronic neuropathic pain such as the gabapentinoids prevents the development of chronic neuropathic pain after surgery is not entirely clear but some studies have shown promising results.

Nerve Growth Factor (NGF)

The experience with development and testing of the NGF blocker, tanezumab, nicely illustrates the positives and the negatives associated with new drug development for chronic pain. As noted in Chap. 7, release of NGF with tissue and nerve injury leads to a cascade of events that cause chronic neuropathic pain. Skin injection of NGF in rodents and humans produces hypersensitivity to pain within a few hours. Based on numerous studies in animals showing that blocking NGF or its receptor TrkA blocks the development of chronic pain, Pfizer pharmaceutical developed a humanized monoclonal antibody, tanazemab, that binds and inhibits NGF and conducted a series of proof-of-concept trials initially focusing on treatment of chronic arthritic pain. In a well publicized placebo controlled trial published in the *New England Journal of Medicine* in 2010 researchers in Canada reported that tanazemab was much better than placebo for treating chronic arthritic pain of the knees. Side effects among tanazemab-treated patients were modest only slightly greater than those among placebo-treated patients. Excitement in the pain community was great and Pfizer began to plan the large definitive trails needed to obtain FDA approval for tanazemab.

However, problems developed over the next few years and in December 2012 the FDA placed a clinical hold on trials using tanazemab and all other anti-NGF antibodies except for trials being conducted for terminal cancer pain. Studies in adult animals identified unexpected damage to the sympathetic nervous system after treatment with tanazemab and longer term human studies found that tanazemab-treated patients required knee replacement surgery sooner than those treated with placebo. The latter observation raised an interesting dilemma. Was the need for earlier surgery due to some unexpected side-effect of the drug or because treated patients had such good relief of pain from the drug that they overused their joints causing greater arthritic damage. Pain serves a warning function and in some circumstances pain suppression can have unexpected consequences (recall the problems faced by patients born insensitive to pain mentioned in Chap. 1).

But the saga of tanazemab was not over. In February 2015 Pfizer submitted extensive animal data on the response of the autonomic nervous system to tanazemab convincing the FDA to reinstate clinical trials. In March 2015 Pfizer announced that they had joined forces with Eli Lilly to conduct a large scale definitive clinical trial on tanazemab. Eli Lilly paid Pfizer $200 million dollars up front as part of their collaborative agreement. If tanazemab makes it through the clinical trials and is approved by the FDA how much will it cost? A similar humanized antibody drug, daclizumab, recently approved by the FDA for treating multiple sclerosis (by blocking a receptor on immune cells) costs about $7500 dollars per dose typically given by injection once a month ($83,000 per year). An estimated 20% of adults suffer from some type of chronic pain so the impact of an effective but costly treatment on the medical system could be enormous. A recent study estimated that the cost per dose would have to be no more than $400 in order for tanazemab to be cost effective for treating chronic pain. How does tanazemab compare with other currently available treatments for chronic pain such as the much cheaper NSAIDs? So far no such comparisons have been made.

Only a subset (about half) of peripheral pain fibers express TrkA receptors (the receptor for NGF) so depending on the innervation pattern, injury to some tissues responds better to NGF blockade than injury to other tissues. Bone and nerve pain seem to be particularly responsive NGF blockers. NGF release with tissue injury activates brain derived nerve growth factor (BDNF) at synapses in the dorsal horn activating its receptor TrkB which appears to be key for inducing central sensitization to pain. Blockers of the BDNF/TrkB signaling pathway are also being developed and they also appear to be effective for treating chronic pain. The ideal drug would be a safe orally administered small molecule that would selectively block TrkA or TrkB. So far none have been identified. Even if such molecules are found there will still be concern about long term effects of blocking NGF and BDNF signaling on tissue repair, neuroendocrine function and brain neurons that are sensitive to NGF and BDNF.

Voltage Gated Ion Channels

Many of the current drugs used to treat chronic neuropathic pain are ion channel blockers (see Chap. 8). The problem is they are nonspecific blockers that have effects throughout the central nervous system. Even the drugs that are specific for certain types of ion channels such as sodium and calcium channels, block a wide range of channel subtypes and have a wide range of effects on the central nervous system. As our understanding of the different subtypes of ion channels has advanced the goal is to develop drugs that selectively block ion channels primarily expressed in the pain pathways or those overexpressed with chronic neuropathic pain.

Sodium Channels

Of the nine sodium channel isoforms (Nav 1.1–1.9) expressed in the nervous system, Nav 1.7, 1.8 and 1.9 are mainly expressed in the dorsal root ganglia and Nav 1.8 is expressed only in the dorsal root ganglia. Mutations in all three of the genes that code for these sodium channels can produce decreased or increased sensitivity to pain depending on the type of mutation (see Chap. 7). Academic and pharmaceutical company researchers have conducted extensive studies in an effort to find selective blockers of these sodium channels over the past few years. Interestingly several of the most promising compounds have been isolated from the venoms of spiders and snails. These venoms contain a range of peptides (a short sequence of amino acids) that work by blocking different subsets of ion channels and receptors thus paralyzing their prey.

As an example of how the process works, researchers at Amgen analyzed tarantula venom and identified 84 different peptides in samples of venom. They tested each peptide for its ability to block Nav 1.7 and compared the blocking ability with other known Nav1.7 peptide blockers. One peptide, named GpTx, was a highly selective blocker of Nav 1.7 and appeared to be a more potent blocker than other previously identified peptides. They identified the aminoacidic sequence of GpTx and then systematically changed amino acids at each position to determine which amino acids were most important for selectivity to Nav 1.7. Finally they tested different aminoacids in each of these positions to arrive at an analog that was more potent and highly selective for Nav 1.7.

As another example researchers at Pfizer started with a compound related to the sodium channel blocker and antiepileptic drug, lamotrigine with the goal of developing a selective orally administered blocker of Nav 1.8. They systematically altered the side chains of the basic backbone of the molecule to arrive at a compound that was a highly selective Nav 1.8 blocker. The compound was effective in several animal models of neuropathic pain without altering normal peripheral or central nervous system function. All of the major pharmaceutical companies are conducting similar research with the goal of finding selective blockers of Nav 1.7, 1.8, and 1.9 and most compounds are still in preclinical animal trials but a few have reached early proof of concept clinical trials in humans.

Calcium Channels

Two of the commonly used current drugs for treating chronic neuropathic pain, gabapentin and pregabalin, are thought to work by blocking a subunit of calcium channels expressed at excitatory synapses throughout the nervous system. N-type calcium channels are more selectively expressed in pain pathways and appear to be better targets for more selective blockage of pain transmission. As noted in Chap. 7, animals with mutations in N-type Cav 2.2 and 3.2 have decreased sensitivity to pain.

In the late 1960s University of Utah biologist, Baldomero Olivera, began reporting on his studies of the venoms of marine cone snails, so-called conotoxins. Olivera was intrigued by tales of the deadly effects of the conotoxins told when he was a child in the Philippines. Some 500 species of marine cone snails produce venoms with up to 200 different peptides that target multiple neurotransmitter receptors and ion channels including several N-type calcium channel blockers. In the early 1980s a young research scientist, Michael McIntosh, joined Olivera in separating out the different conotoxins and they identified a potent N-type calcium channel blocker, ziconotide. Animal studies showed it was very effective for treating chronic neuropathic pain and it was manufactured into an artificial drug called Prialt by Elan Corporation. The FDA gave approval for use in December, 2004. Although ziconotide has been remarkably effective for treating severe chronic pain its use has been mainly limited to treating terminal cancer patients because it can only be safely administered by injection directly into the spinal fluid. Efforts are underway to improve the delivery of ziconotide and related conotoxins and to develop better small molecule N-type calcium channel blockers that can be administered orally.

Transient Receptor Potential (TRP) Receptors

As described in Chap. 2, TRP receptors are expressed by afferent pain fibers where they detect a variety of noxious stimuli including temperature and acidic conditions. Mutations in the gene that codes for TRPA1 cause a familial episodic pain syndrome. TRPV1 is activated by capsaicin, an ingredient in chili peppers. The fact that capsaicin is used for pain relief in a variety of liniments and ointments may seem like a paradox since activating TRPV1 channels causes increased firing of the afferent pain fibers (see Chap. 4). Indeed when capsaicin is placed on the skin it initially causes burning pain but with time the burning disappears and the area becomes less sensitive to pain as the TRPV1 channels become desensitized. By applying a local anesthetic to the painful area prior to topical application of capsaicin the initial burning pain can be prevented. Several small molecules that block TRPV1 were developed at the beginning of this century and several reached early phase clinical trials but enthusiasm diminished when they were found to adversely effect the core body temperature. Glenmark developed a TRPA1 blocker, GRC17536 that was shown to be significantly better than placebo in early clinical trials for treating diabetic peripheral neuropathy. Several other TRP blockers are in early stage clinical trials.

Opioids

The holly grail in the quest for better pain treatment is a new opioid drug without the bothersome side effects and the addiction potential of traditional opioid drugs. Past experience has taught us to be wary of claims for such a drug without having data on long term follow up of treated patients. Researchers at Stanford University and the University of California at San Francisco claim that they may have found the holly grail in a compound called PZM21. To find the compound they first made a detailed 3D structural model of the binding site of the most important opioid receptor for pain transmission. Using computers they tested in excess of three million compounds each with an average of over a million configurations to identify compounds that best fit the binding site. They gradually whittled down the number of compounds to three based on further testing. They then tested 500 analogs of the three narrowing the field to 15, then seven and finally one. They then manipulated the molecules in this compound to get the absolute best possible fit to the opioid receptor binding site, ending up with PZM21.

When they gave PZM21 to mice it provided comparable pain relief as morphine and the relief lasted longer than comparable doses of morphine. They assessed pain by measuring how long mice would tolerate standing on a hot surface. The mice given PZM21 were no more likely to return to the place where they received the drug than to a similar chamber where they could receive salt solution so there was no sign of addiction. Equally important the mice that received PZM21 developed fewer side effects than morphine including the bothersome constipation and respiratory depression. Of course the key question is how PZM21 will work in humans and proof-of-concept trials are underway.

Cannabinoids

The cannibinoid receptors and endogenous transmitters along with their metabolizing enzymes make up the endocannabinoid system (ECS), a "hot" target for new pain drug development. The ECS interacts with other endogenous pain control systems particularly the opioid system at multiple levels and is active at both excitatory and inhibitory synapses.

As with new onset pain, smoked cannabis or ingestion of its main active ingredient, THC has not been very effective for treating chronic pain in several controlled treatment trials. Drugs combining THC with other minor components of cannabis have produced better results in treatment trials for chronic pain. Cannabidiol (CBD) in particular moderates the psychoactive effects of THC and seems to improve the analgesic effects. One compound in particular, Sativex marketed by GW Pharmaceuticals has shown promise in treating chronic neuropathic pain. Sativex, which is administered as an oral-mucosal spray, combines THC and CBD in a 1:1 ratio along with several other minor cannabis substances. Initial treatment trials with Sativex have shown good results for treating a variety of chronic pain disorders with much less intoxication than seen with THC compounds. Sativex was approved in Canada for treating chronic neuropathic pain associated with multiple sclerosis in 2005 and for treating chronic cancer pain in 2007. It is currently on the fast track for approval by the FDA in the United States for treating chronic cancer pain. Initial treatment trials of Sativex for treating both peripheral and central neuropathic pain produced promising results.

An example of the complexities and risks involved in drug development is illustrated in a recent phase 1 treatment trial of a new cannabinoid drug for neuropathic pain carried out in France. In phase 1 trials the main goal is to determine drug safety with only secondary interest is efficacy. Phase 2 trials focus on efficacy but typically are not large enough to be definitive whereas phase 3 trials are large enough to be definitive. Drug companies typically must have results from all three phases to obtain approval for sale of a new drug. The drug called BIA 10-2474 was intended to target the ECS and inhibit neuropathic pain. In the trial six young healthy volunteers received 50 mg of BIA 10-2474 and two received placebo. The drug was administered for 6 days and all six subjects who received the drug developed neuro-logical symptoms with onset from day 5 on the drug to 2 days after receiving the drug. One subject died and at least two others have severe permanent neurological dysfunction (some of the data has still not been released). The drug company, Bial of Portugal indicated that preliminary studies in animals and in human subjects showed no similar toxicity but presumably the human subjects did not receive the drug for 6 days (again details were not released). The final conclusion was that although the drug was meant to target the ECS unidentified "off-target" effects must have occurred.

Glutamate

As noted in Chap. 8, release of the excitatory neurotransmitter glutamate at the dorsal horn primary pain neuron synapses, is key to development of central hyper-sensitivity to pain after nerve injury. The second order transmission neurons and interneurons express several different glutamate receptors but the most important for developing pain hypersensitivity are the AMPA and NMDA receptors. Drugs that block AMPA or NMDA receptors prevent the development of central sensitiza-tion to pain after nerve injury but since there are multiple subtypes of these recep-tors and different subtypes are expressed throughout the central nervous system side effects are common, particularly sedation and memory impairment. For example the AMPA receptor blocker, NBQX, is a better sedative than a pain medication. The potent NMDA blocker, ketamine produces a trance-like state, sedation and memory loss after intravenous injection. A less potent NMDA receptor blocker, dextro-methorphan, is widely available in over-the-counter cough medications but has not been very useful for management of chronic pain. Ifenprodil and traxoprodil are newer NMDA receptor blockers and traxoprodil has entered clinical trials for treat-ing chronic neuropathic pain.

Gamma-Aminobutyric Acid (GABA)

GABA is the main inhibitory neurotransmitter within the central pain pathways and drugs that enhance GABA neurotransmission (GABA agonists) tend to suppress the development of chronic pain. However, as in the case of the glutamate receptors, there are two major classes of GABA receptors, $GABA_A$ and $GABA_B$ and each has multiple subtypes with different functions. For example, $GABA_A$ subtypes have dif-ferent anxiolytic, sedative, amnestic and analgesic effects. Activating the α_1 subtype produces sedation while activating the α_2 and α_3 subtypes produce anxiolytic and analgesic effects. The commonly used GABA agonists, diazepam (Valium) and midazolam (Versed), activate multiple receptor subtypes producing a combination of effects including sedation and pain suppression. This combination of effects is useful when a drug such as midazolam is used for minor surgical procedures but is a major drawback when the drug is used to treat chronic pain. Merck and Company developed a drug called L- 838,417 that selectively activates the α_2 and α_3 receptors producing anxiolytic and analgesic effects without sedation in rodents. Whether the drug will have the same effect in humans is being evaluated.

Noradrenalin

As described in Chap. 8, neurons containing noradrenalin located in the locus cerelius (LC) influence pain transmission in the spinal cord and brain. Of the different noradrenalin receptor subtypes, the α_2 receptor is most important for pain transmission particularly in the spinal cord where drugs that activate α_2 receptors inhibit pain transmission and drugs that block α_2 receptors enhance pain transmission. By contrast, activating α_1 receptors enhances pain transmission in the spinal cord. Clonidine, a selective α_2 receptor agonist, commonly used for treating hypertension, has also been used to treat chronic pain. When combined with local anesthetics, steroids or opioids, epidural or intradural injections enhance the degree and duration of pain control in a variety of patients with chronic pain. In one small controlled treatment trial a single dose of oral clonidine 2 h before hysterectomy surgery significantly decreased postoperative pain compared to placebo. Clonidine does have many potential side effects including drops in blood pressure and rapid heart beats and there are many potential drug interactions so that use of clonidine for pain control has been limited. Noradrenalin potentiates the effect of opioids in treating chronic pain probably through the α_2 receptors. Noradrenergic agonists and reuptake inhibitors enhance the analgesic effects of opioids. As noted in Chap. 4, weaker opioid drugs such as tramadol activate both opioid and noradrenalin receptors. Selective α_2 receptor agonists, ST-91 and UK 14,304 have been effective for pain relief in animal models but so far have not been evaluated in human clinical trials.

Dopamine

Interest in the use of dopamine agonists for treating chronic pain has increased in recent years as understanding of central dopamine pathways has advanced (see Chap. 8). Unlike most other drugs discussed in this chapter, drugs that modulate dopamine (dopamine agonists) not only block pain transmission but also play a complex role in the motivational-emotional component of pain. Brain dopamine levels correlate with the magnitude of perceived pain rather than the magnitude of the painful stimulus. There is convincing evidence that the decreased motivation seen in patients with chronic pain is due to decreased levels of dopamine. Furthermore, as noted in Chap. 8, there is a complex relationship between the dopamine motivational/reward network and the response to opioid drugs. With chronic pain the reward effect of opioids is diminished. Pramipexole, a dopamine agonist that mainly activates D_3 receptors, was initially developed to treat Parkinson disease but later found to be effective for treating restless leg syndrome and chronic pain. Controlled treatment trials found it to be effective for treating fibromyalgia, a chronic generalized pain disorder of unknown cause that has been relatively refractory to other pain medications. Anecdotal reports suggest pramipexole may be useful for treating chronic neuropathic pain but so far there have been no controlled treatment trials.

Targeted Drug Delivery

Rather than developing a drug that is specific for pain transmission another strategy to avoid unwanted systemic side effects is to deliver a drug to a localized region within the pain transmission pathways. The dorsal root ganglia (DRG) is an appealing target since it contains only primary sensory neurons and is relatively easy to reach via a needle passed through the bony foramen where the spinal nerve exits the spine. As noted in Chap. 2, the DRG is located between the dorsal root and the spinal nerve and pain sensing neurons in the DRG contribute to chronic pain with increased excitability and spontaneous firing. The DRG lacks a protective capsular membrane and has a rich density of capillaries so that it is readily permeable to drugs yet resistant to toxic concentrations because of the high blood perfusion rate. Furthermore, the DRG lacks the neurovascular barrier (blood brain barrier) that is present throughout the central nervous system so that large molecules and even cells injected into the region of the DRG easily diffuse into the ganglia.

In rats who have undergone a selective ligation of a lumbar spinal nerve (a popular model for studying sciatica), a single injection of steroids near the DRG attenuates the development of hypersensitivity, reduces sympathetic sprouting, reduces nerve growth factor release and decreases microglial activation in the spinal cord. Injection of selective sodium and calcium channel blockers into the DRG prevents the development of chronic pain. As described in Chap. 4, injecting steroids (along with a local anesthetic) into the epidural space is a common treatment for patients with new onset sciatica. The drugs make their way to the DRG but in much lower concentrations that could be achieved with a selective DRG injection. Some studies in patients with sciatica suggest that selective DRG injections may be better than epidural injections but definitive controlled treatment comparison trials are not available. Physicians require extensive training to perform localized DRG injections so such injections are only available in specialized clinics. The DRG is reached by guiding a needle through the intervertebral foramen using radiographic imaging. Whether steroids or any other drugs applied to the DRG in patients can prevent development of chronic sciatica is currently unknown.

Even more promising than targeted delivery of drugs for treating chronic sciatica is the targeted delivery of stem cells or viral vectors to permanently modify pain transmission. Again the DRG is an ideal target because of its lack of a protective capsule and its rich vascular supply. Preliminary studies in the spinal nerve ligation rat model of sciatica suggest that injecting stem cells derived from bone marrow into the DRG prevents the development of chronic pain. The stem cells are taken up by the DRG and are distributed around the primary pain neurons resembling glial cells. These "satellite cells" secrete several molecules that prevent the development of central sensitization and the development of chronic pain. In the same rat model of sciatica, investigators found that injecting recombinant adeno-associated virus into the DRG prevents the development of chronic sciatica after nerve injury. The virus carried a transgene that codes for a peptide that blocks the Cav 2.2 N-type calcium channel key in pain transmission. The advantages of this type of targeted therapy are that the channel blockage only occurs in the sensory neurons of the DRG and the effect is long-lasting and may even be permanent.

Targeted Stimulation and Ablation Procedures

As noted in Chap. 8, nerve and brain stimulation and ablation procedures are becoming more popular for treating chronic pain as our ability to produce localized stimulation and ablation has advanced with new microelectrode and image guiding techniques. This technology will continue to advance but there is a critical need for controlled treatment trials to identify the most effective stimulus parameters (magnitude, frequency and duration of electrical stimulation) and the long term benefit and risks with localized ablation. Even with the technological advances for inserting a fine needle or tiny probe into nerves and brain, these are still relatively crude procedures with major potential risks. The soft nerve and brain tissues are easily damaged and the immune system tries to isolate foreign bodies by surrounding them with scar tissue.

The future of targeted stimulation and ablation procedures lies with nanoparticle technology. Tiny molecules that recognize a specific protein such as an ion channel or receptor can be injected into the blood stream where they make their way to their target. Molecules that stimulate or damage neurons can be attached to antibodies or other molecules that recognize a selective target within the pain pathways. For example, researchers at the MIT developed a tiny ferromagnetic particle that targets the primary pain receptor TRPV1 (see Chap. 2). This receptor that is present in primary pain nerve endings, senses heat and the chemical capsaicin. The ferromagnetic particles generate localized heat when exposed to an electromagnetic field that in turn activates the TRPV1 channel and triggers firing. This technology is already being used to selectively target malignant cells in brain cancer but there are still many problems to overcome before these procedures reach the pain clinic.

Overview

Treatment of chronic neuropathic pain, chronic sciatica in particular, is one of the most challenging problems in modern clinical neurology. In order to develop better treatments we need to better understand the relationship between symptoms and pain mechanisms. Recent advances in our understanding of peripheral and central pain hypersensitization after nerve injury have identified molecular mechanisms for possible intervention but we are still in the early stages of developing and testing new treatments. The cost of developing and conducting clinical trials of new treatments is a major limiting factor.

Suggested Additional Reading

Bornini S, Rase G. Editorial: first in-human trials – what we can learn from tragic failures. N Engl J Med. 2016;375:1786–9.

Crile GW. The kinetic theory of shock and its prevention through anoci-association (shockless operation). Lancet. 1913;182:7–16.

Lane NE, Schnitzer TJ, Birbara CA, et al. Tanezumab for treatment of pain from osteoarthritis of the knee. N Engl J Med. 2010;363:1521–31.

Manglik A, Lin H, Aryal DK, et al. Structure-based discovery of opioid analgesics with reduced side effects. Nature. 2016;537:185–90.

Rahn EJ, Hohmann AG. Cannabinoids as pharmacotherapies for neuropathic pain: from the bench to the bedside. Neurotherapeeutics. 2009;6:713–37.

Chapter 10
Some Final Thoughts

Nearly everyone experiences back pain at sometime in their life and up to 5% have sciatica. Yet how patients are diagnosed and managed varies greatly depending on where they are and what physician they see. Primary care physicians, including family practice and emergency room physicians, have largely become triage officers referring patients with sciatica to specialists for management. If you are referred to a neurologist you will likely be given pain medication and probably a course of physical therapy, if you are referred to an orthopedic surgeon or neurosurgeon there is a better chance you will have surgery, if you are referred to a spine clinic you likely will receive epidural steroid injections, and if you are referred to a chiropractor you will have a series of manipulations. The referral patterns vary from physician to physician and in different parts of the country. Worldwide the United States has the highest rate of surgery for low back pain and sciatica. Patients in the United States are five times more likely to have surgery than patients in the United Kingdom. If patients have insurance, they will usually have routine x-rays and an MRI of the low back often before being referred to a specialist. These are expensive procedures that often lead to equivocal results (such as the ubiquitous degenerative disc disease). As noted earlier, evidence based guidelines recommend initial conservative management of patients with sciatica unless there are "red flags" on the clinical evaluation. Most patients will get better within 6 weeks. This means no laboratory tests and no treatment other than pain management and encouragement to resume normal activities as much as possible.

Who identifies the "red flags?" This is a problem. Most primary care physicians don't feel confident evaluating patients with sciatica for "red flags". This requires a detailed neurological history and examination and most primary care physicians have little if any neurological training. In addition, it takes time, at least half an hour and usually longer, and the current medical system does not reward physician time spent talking with and examining patients. Neurologists are trained to evaluate patients with back pain and sciatica, but traditionally, in this country, they see only a small percentage of these patients. There is a general frustration that not much can be done. Primary care physicians often use the MRI as a substitute for a time

© Springer International Publishing AG, part of Springer Nature 2019

R. W. Baloh, *Sciatica and Chronic Pain*,
https://doi.org/10.1007/978-3-319-93904-9_10

consuming clinical evaluation. They rationalize that patients have come to expect high tech testing and that they may be legally vulnerable if they don't get the test. However, patients complain that their doctors do not take time to listen to them. This is why nontraditional medical practitioners are taking over the primary care of many patients with back pain and sciatica.

How can we fix the system that currently is not working for patients with back pain and sciatica? First, we need to convince physicians and patients that a scientific approach using *evidence*-based medicine is in everyone's best interest. This will not be easy. As we have seen, there is a rich tradition of *belief*-based medicine in the United States. A major difficulty with practicing evidence-based medicine in patients with back pain and sciatica is the paucity of well-controlled studies. These studies are difficult to organize, are very expensive to conduct, and typically take years to complete. In the past, there were no imaging techniques to document nerve compression so the diagnosis was always in doubt. MRI has changed everything and with current technology, it is possible to visualize the spinal nerves and the entire sciatic nerve. But should every patient with sciatica undergo an MRI of the low back and pelvis (with neurography to look for nerve damage and with contrast to rule out tumors)? Can we afford it? The answer is no to both questions, but we can afford to design and perform well-controlled studies using MRI. These would have to be supported by the government. The National Institute of Health (NIH) has the necessary resources and says it's committed to translational research – bringing scientific discoveries to clinical practice.

In the meantime, guidelines for management of patients with back pain and sciatica have to be based on current evidence. Overall, patients can be reassured that their prognosis is good even though some will have persistent or recurrent symptoms. There is broad consensus that bed rest should be discouraged and that patients should be advised to stay active and gradually increase their activity level. If their pain is so severe that bed rest is required, the goal is to get the patient out of bed as soon as possible (usually no more than a few days). There is general consensus for the concept of "red flags" to identify patients who require imaging of the low back and referral to a specialist. As for pain medications, acetaminophen and NSAIDs are the consensus first line choices and other drugs such as muscle relaxants, opioids, and compound medications (acetaminophen and hydromorphone, acetaminophen and tramadol) are second line choices. Long-term regular use of opioids or any other pain medication should be avoided. Over prescribing of opioids for back pain and sciatica is a major contributor to the current opioid crisis in the United States. With chronic neuropathic pain regular daily use of pain medications may actually aggravate the problem. In this case medications that stabilize damaged nerves such as antiepileptic and antidepressant drugs are more useful. Newer more selective medications for acute and chronic pain are in the pipeline of development but based on past experience early claims of efficacy should be viewed with caution.

Will primary care physicians and patients buy into rigorous guidelines for management of sciatica? Currently most primary care physicians are either unaware of or disagree with the management guidelines for sciatica. Patients usually rely on their physician to make diagnostic and therapeutic decisions, but they want information so they can be involved in the decision process. Of course some completely bypass traditional medicine and go directly to a chiropractor or other nontraditional therapists. The danger here is that treatment is given without a diagnosis. Subluxation is not a diagnosis to explain sciatica. No doubt "the laying on of hands" is a powerful treatment, but if the patient has a tumor or some other structural damage proper diagnosis and appropriate treatment are delayed. Educating physicians and patients will be a difficult process.

I can't overemphasize the importance of a well-trained, caring physician in this equation. Guidelines are just that, a roadmap to help physicians develop a management strategy. The guidelines emphasize the importance of a careful history and examination and that takes time and as noted earlier, the current system does not reward physicians who spend the necessary time to perform a careful history and examination. In my experience of over 40 years of seeing patients, it takes at least 30 min to perform an adequate history and examination, think through the problem, and formulate a plan of action. This does not include the time needed to review records and generate a report. And this is an "intense" 30 min that can be repeated at most 8–10 times a day. I am literally exhausted after such a day. I can't imagine how some physicians see 30–40 patients a day, 5–6 days a week. Clearly, they can't properly evaluate so many patients in 1 day. A common solution is to order tests and treat symptoms without a diagnosis. Chiropractors have the ultimate solution – they know the diagnosis in advance: subluxation of a vertebra. They take an x-ray that confirms it and they spend their time treating the patient with the "laying on of hands." This approach works reasonably well for back pain since the vast majority of patients have minor musculoskeletal damage and will get better in a few weeks regardless of what is done. There is even the occasional patient where one of the lateral articulations of the vertebrae are caught in an unusual position and held in that position by muscle spasm. Manipulations followed by an audible snap or pop as the lateral articulation returns to its normal position leads to a dramatic cure and the kind of testimonial that assures a steady flow of patients. But this approach does not work with sciatica. Patients with nerve compression can have worsening of symptoms and signs after manipulation. Even if not, the diagnosis is delayed and more appropriate treatment withheld.

To replace "belief" based medicine with "evidence" based medicine, we will need major changes in how medical services are rewarded. The difficult task of talking to a patient and applying scientific based evidence to solve their problems needs to be rewarded at a higher level. Medicare and medical insurance companies have addressed the problem of reimbursement inequities over the past 15 years but the resulting changes have only been cosmetic. There is still a strong bias toward rewarding tests and procedures. Time spent doing tests and procedures is rewarded 3–10 times greater than time spent talking to patients. Specialties such as neurology and pediatrics where the majority of time is spent evaluating and managing patient problems have seen a steady decline in reimbursements while specialties such as radiology and surgery where the majority of time is spent doing procedures have had a steady increase in reimbursements. Not surprisingly the number of applicants for neurology and pediatric residencies are steadily declining. The inertia of the current system is so great that I don't see the needed changes coming in the near future. A few years ago a large group of Neurologists visited Capital Hill to discuss their concerns about low reimbursement rates for cognitive services at a time when there was increasing demand for such services. They did not receive much encouragement. If anything the atmosphere has gotten worse and the gridlock in congress has increased.

The risk of continuing on the current path is that alternative belief-based medical treatments will continue to thrive and even grow in prominence. BJ Palmer, the son of the founder of chiropractic DD Palmer, laid down the gauntlet for the medical community in 1919 when he said:

> "Give me a simple mind that thinks along simple tracts, give me 30 days to instruct him, and that individual can go forth on the highways and byways and get more sick people well than the best, most complete, all around, unlimited medical education of any medical man that ever lived." (quoted from: Homola S. Chiropractic. *Clin Orthop Rel Dis*. 2006;444:236)

Suggested Additional Reading

DeVocht JW. History and overview of theories and methods of chiropractic: a counterpoint. Clin Orthop Relat Res. 2006;444:236–42.

Homola S. Chiropractic. Clin Orthop Rel Dis. 2006;444:236.

Hopayian K, Notley C. A systematic review of low back pain and sciatica patients' expectations and experience of health care. Spine J. 2014;14:1769–80.

Webster BS, Courtney TK, Huang Y-H, et al. Physicians' initial management of acute back pain versus evidence-based guidelines. J Gen Intern Med. 2005;20:1132–5.

Index